# INDEPENDENT LIVING

# INDEPENDENT LIVING

## Philosophy, Process, and Services

*Charlene P. DeLoach*, Ph.D.
*Ronnie D. Wilkins*, Ed.D.
*Guy W. Walker*, M.Ed.
*Department of Special Education and Rehabilitation,*
*Memphis State University*

*University Park Press* • BALTIMORE

*UNIVERSITY PARK PRESS*
*International Publishers in Medicine and Human Services*
*300 North Charles Street*
*Baltimore, Maryland 21201*

*Copyright © 1983 by University Park Press*

*Manufactured in the United States of America by The Maple Press Company*

**Library of Congress Cataloging in Publication Data**

DeLoach, Charlene.
  Independent living.

  Includes index.
  1. Handicapped—United States—Life skills guides.  2. Rehabilitation—United States.  I. Wilkins, Ronnie D. II. Walker, Guy W. III. Title.
HV1553.D445  1983     362.4'0483     82–21949
ISBN 0–8391–1794–9

# Contents

**v**

PART TWO *Essential Support Services*

# Preface

This text evolved from the authors' attempts to define and clarify for their students and themselves this complex social services delivery concept of independent living. In the larger society independent living is an expected and comparatively easy goal to obtain. In the normal course of events an infant learns first to walk, then to eat, and then to dress independently, and while still a child he or she begins to make decisions about where to walk, what foods to eat, and what type of clothing to wear. In the normal course of events self-care skills develop naturally and evolve into self-determining behaviors.

Independent living as a social service paradigm, however, concerns itself with the development of these skills and these behaviors when the course of events is not normal. Some people, because of disability, are not able to develop these independent living skills and behaviors to the same extent or at the same pace as an able-bodied person. In other cases the ability to live independently may be lost because of disability or because of the functional limitations sometimes associated with old age. The process of independent living rehabilitation is thus directed at enabling individuals to acquire or to reacquire those independent living skills in spite of severely handicapping conditions.

The authors recognize that discussing independent living for both elderly disabled people and younger disabled people involves some risk of offending either one or both groups. Some people who are old do not think of themselves as disabled, and do not like being associated with disabled people, even though they may be handicapped by such physical limitations as failing eyesight, poor hearing, chronic cardiovascular conditions, limited mobility due to arthritic joints, and a variety of other disorders. And many young disabled adults resent being associated with elderly people despite the commonality of some of the physical restrictions faced by both groups. However, the authors' intent in this text is to point out that both groups often face similar problems, to remind the reader that many disabled people are old, to suggest that disabled elderly people should be considered legitimate and deserving recipients of independent living services, and yet also to recognize those valid differences between younger and older disabled people which must be considered in the overall philosophies and treatment strategies of independent living service agencies.

Founded on the ground-breaking rehabilitation legislation of the previous decade, independent living as a social service paradigm came of age in the early 1980s. The evolution of this system of rehabilitation services stemmed from several deep-seated societal changes, including high levels of unemployment; increased numbers of disabled people who survived the acute phase of medical care; a growing proportion of people with degenerative disabilities, including many past retirement age; and the burgeoning of improved rehabilitation techniques and innovative adaptive devices. For elderly disabled people, independent living was designed to be a human services system that would allow them to "age in place"—to live out their lives in their own homes or, at least, in their own neighborhoods, where they could continue to enjoy the friends, parks, shops, and streets that were familiar to them. For younger disabled people, independent living was designed to be the human services system that would allow them to be assimilated into and contribute to the general community.

What began as a humanitarian system for improving the quality of the lives of those who were nearing the end of their life spans or were dependent in some area of their basic living needs became, eventually, an economic necessity. With the elimination of federal housing subsidies, with Medicaid regulations that sponsored nursing-home care only for the "sickest of the sick," and with deinstitutionalization policies that reduced the residential populations of institutions for people with physical or mental disabilities, independent living services assumed a major role in fostering the continued survival of disabled people in an increasingly penurious society.

Independent living rehabilitation as a social service system was initiated at a time when the role of government in providing basic human services was being reexamined. This timing jeopardized the very existence of the system, which has the potential to enrich, both now and in the future, the lives of the disabled. Thrust immediately into the position of having to coordinate or directly provide essential services, such as housing, transportation, attendant care, training in basic living skills, and so on, fledgling independent living programs faced the challenge of deciding what services should be rendered and who should receive them. Lacking the expertise that only years of experience can provide, independent living professionals were forced to learn while in the process of providing essential, sometimes lifesaving, services.

In the following pages, the growth of independent living will be traced from its emergence as a social service concept to its culmination as a social service delivery system that assists clients through a variety of delivery formats. Part One describes the evolution of independent living as a social service paradigm and as a cost-effective, humanitarian approach to the living needs of elderly and disabled people. Part Two covers, first, the different people who require rehabilitation-related services in order to attain optimum levels of independent functioning and, second, the contribution of various community-based service providers to these goals. Part Three explains the different modes of independent living and the methods for matching individuals' social and physical competencies with the services, devices, and training required to bring them up to and maintain them at their highest feasible levels of independent functioning. Finally, Part Four explores the external and internal factors that are integral to the success or failure of different types of independent living programs.

Independent living, which has always been the underlying rationale of established models of rehabilitative services, such as medical rehabilitation and vocational rehabilitation, has now been legitimized as a rehabilitation model in its own right. Independent living rehabilitation, which incorporates and enhances the effectiveness of other rehabilitation models, has the potential to help greater numbers of people because it can offer essential services to people of all ages and with all degrees of physical or mental impairments. It is hoped that this text, by establishing a sound theoretical basis for independent living rehabilitation and by describing various means by which theory can be translated into effective modes of delivering specific independent living services, will prove useful as a source book both for professionals and for professionals-in-training.

The authors wish to acknowledge the valuable assistance received from Fred Dinwiddie, director of the Center for Independent Living, Memphis, Tennessee. His knowledge of the current "state of the art" in independent living was helpful to us as we decided how best to present the major models of independent living programs. We also express our thanks to Doug Rice of the Arkansas Rehabilitation Research and Training Center. His careful reading and constructive criticisms of the preliminary manuscript have made this a much stronger work.

Charlene P. DeLoach
Ronnie D. Wilkins
Guy W. Walker

# PART ONE

*Independent Living—*
*Some Basic Concepts*

# 1

# The Evolution of Independent Living as a Human Services Goal

Over three hundred years ago people began to move from Europe to the North American continent. Many of those early settlers came because they wanted more freedom, which is another way of saying that they wanted to be independent. They wanted to independently choose the place, time, and manner of their worship. They also wanted independence from societal forces that severely restricted their economic opportunities. In other words, they wanted to freely choose how they would earn their living, and if they were frugal and industrious they wanted to believe that they would prosper. For centuries people from all over the world continued to come to America in hopes of finding prosperity and independence.

In America, perhaps more than anywhere else, personal freedom and independence have long been principles deemed worthy of defending. Yet here, as elsewhere, people also seem to recognize that no one is completely independent. All people are to some degree interdependent; at times we all need each other.

This interdependence, however, is in no way threatening as long as it does not unreasonably interfere with our individual freedom and right to choose for ourselves in such basic issues as where we will work, live, go to school, attend church, shop, and play. It is that ability to make choices, within reasonable limits, that protects the time-honored principle of independence.

When one is in need of help because of disability, unemployment, or any other reason, one's ability to freely choose is often impaired. The unemployed laborer can choose only the job that happens to be available; the severely disabled person can choose only the school or home that happens to be accessible. These and other constraints imposed by human needs rob us of our independence by simply taking away our choices, and thus one of the most basic responses that human service agencies can make to human needs is to help return that independence by restoring those choices. This text is intended to reveal to the reader how the choices of severely disabled people are restricted and thus how they are robbed of their independence. More importantly, it is intended to explain the many ways in which human service agencies as well as the disabled person himself can restore those choices through the process known as independent living rehabilitation (ILR).

The purposes of Chapter 1 are

1. to define and clarify certain terms that will be used throughout this text,

2. to discuss the evolution of the concept of independent living rehabilitation, and

3. to relate the contribution of a number of different social and human service programs to the development of the concept of independent living rehabilitation.

## DEFINITION OF TERMS

In this section five terms will be defined and discussed. The first three of these, "disability," "handicap," and "elderly," are used in identifying those people who receive independent living (IL) services. The other two, "rehabilitation" and "independent living rehabilitation" (ILR), are used in describing the process of delivering IL services. The terms are discussed beyond mere definitions, for it is important to understand that they are not necessarily used in this text in the way that one often hears them used in everyday language.

The first terms to be discussed are disability and handicap. These two terms are often used interchangeably, but important distinctions are made between them in this text.

## DISABILITY

Hamilton (1950, p. 17) gave definitions of both disability and handicap that have been widely used and that offer an appropriate beginning point for understanding these terms. Disability, Hamilton says, is "a condition of impairment, physical or mental, having an objective aspect that can usually be described by a physician." This definition has been generally agreed upon and further developed by subsequent authors such as B. A. Wright (1960), Rubin and Roessler (1978), and G. N. Wright (1980). With this definition as a guide, four points will be made that will help in understanding disability and that will also help in comparing disability with handicap later.

First, a disability has an "objective aspect," in contrast to a handicap, which is relative in nature. B. A. Wright (1960) points out that a disability is "more particularly a medical condition, whereas a handicap more nearly refers to the somatopsychological relationship" (p. 9). In more pragmatic terms, one might better understand the objective nature of a disability by thinking of its resulting limitations. For example, if two people both have a complete lesion of the spinal cord at the sixth cervical vertebra as a disability, the objective nature of disability will mean (among other things) that the degree of physical impairment caused by the disability will be much the same for both. There may be minor differences because of slight differences in the injuries or other physical characteristics of the people, but the physical limitations resulting from the disability will be more alike than different. In terms of physical functioning, it will not matter if one person is highly educated and the other is not, if one is employed and the other is not, or if one is wealthy and the other is not.

The second important point is that disability is a "condition" resulting from illness, injury, or congenital causes. Often people equate disability with illness. This unfortunate error contributes to many myths and stereotypes about those who are disabled. For example, an uninformed employer might refuse to hire a disabled applicant because he equates disability with sickness and expects an excessive amount of absenteeism and unusual health care needs from the applicant. Or, from a social perspective, friends and acquaintances might have unnecessary reservations about a disabled person's ability to participate in a wide range of social activities. These examples illustrate the negative reactions that people sometimes have to a disabled person, partly because they incorrectly assume that the disability implies that some active disease is present. Disability should be understood as an ongoing condition that is a result of an injury, illness, or congenital cause.

Third, a disability can usually be verified, described, or diagnosed by a physician or other appropriate professional. This is related to the objective nature of disability, for, in theory at least, a competent physician can arrive at an accurate diagnosis of a disability if presented with adequate information. This is still true for mental and emotional disabilities, even though the diagnostic procedures may be less precise than with most physical disorders.

Finally, a disability limits or impairs physical or mental functioning. A person with a disability will have functional limitations, and these limitations are used as a means of describing the effect of the disability upon the person. For example, inability to walk because of paralysis is a functional limitation resulting from a level C6 spinal cord injury. In the case of mental or emotional disability, the functional limitation may be an inability to make accurate judgments based on subjective information, an inability to respond appropriately in various social situations, or an inability to use abstract reasoning. It is the functional limitation resulting from the disability that becomes a barrier to a person in reaching his or her goals in life, and thus it is the functional limitation that provides the bridge from the term disability to the term handicap. Here the two terms overlap.

## HANDICAP

Hamilton (1950) defined handicap as "the cumulative result of the obstacles which disability interposes between the individual and his maximum functional level" (p. 17). B. A. Wright (1960) and Rubin and Roessler (1978) have used this definition without any change, but G. N. Wright (1980) points out that it does not adequately distinguish between handicap and disability. He states that a handicap is "a disadvantage, interference, or barrier to performance, opportunity, or fulfillment in any desired role in life (e.g., vocational, social, educational, familial), imposed upon the individual by limitation in function or by other problems associated with disability and/or personal characteristics in the context of the individual's environment or role" (p. 68). Thus, Wright correctly recognizes handicap as a much broader concept than disability.

In the discussion of handicap, as with disability, several points will be stressed. G. N. Wright's definition will be used as a guide.

First, Wright states that a handicap is the result of an accumulation of factors. The factors that can handicap a person certainly include disability, but they are not limited to it. Earlier it was noted that disability overlaps with handicap in that a disability results in functional limitations. These functional limitations represent the handicap imposed by a disability. That is, a person with the disability of spinal cord injury is functionally impaired (that is, handicapped) in that he or she is unable to stand and walk. That person, however, might also be handicapped by a number of other factors such as, age, education, work experience, sex, race, or even the geographic location of his or her home. It is important to note that any factor that can handicap a person can take on new significance when that factor is joined by a disability. For example, a person without a high-school education is to some degree handicapped in the job market, but add to that handicap the additional handicap of a disability such as quadriplegia and the educational limitation has a much greater impact than before. Furthermore, add advanced age to the other two handicaps and this hypothetical person has probably lost all hope of finding employment. Such combinations of handicaps seem to be multiplicative rather than additive in terms of the problems they present to the individual.

Second, a person may be handicapped or prevented from functioning effectively in more than one life role or area. For example, a person handicapped by a respiratory disease may be severely limited in his usual job role (for example, farmer). He may be limited in one area of personal interest (for example, participation in athletic events) but not in another (for example, reading or playing chess). Finally, he may not be limited at all in his familial role of husband and father. Thus, handicaps may affect different life roles to greater and lesser degrees.

This leads directly to the third point, which is that handicap is a relative term. A specific impairment will have a different effect upon different people because other aspects of their lives differ. For example, imagine two men named Jim and Woody, each of whom has the disability of a spinal cord injury at the sixth cervical vertebra (that is, a level C6 injury). As stated earlier their functional limitations will be generally the same, but they are handicapped in quite different ways. Before their disabilities Jim's favorite pastime was playing softball on a church team, and Woody's favorite pastime was designing and playing computer games. Jim has worked all his adult life as a brickmason. Woody has worked as a computer programming instructor in a community college. Jim is 51 years old, and Woody is 33. Given these brief descriptions, it is clear that the extent of their handicaps is quite different. Jim will need to make major changes in his occupation and recreational activity, and his age may be a handicap to him in making those changes, especially the occupational ones. On the other hand, Woody may well be able to continue his current job and hobby with only minor adjustments.

The preceding discussion leads to the conclusion that the severity of a given handicap varies from person to person and from situation to situation. This is the most important point regarding this concept. It is here that one can most appreciate the distinction between handicap and disability. A disability will impose the same functional limitations upon a person at work, at home, in a park, or in a shopping center, but the degree to which those functional limitations impair the person's ability to accomplish his or her objectives in each of those places will likely be quite different in each situation.

For independent living, the significance of the distinction between disability and handicap is clear. Severe disabilities will impose functional limitations that may result in major problems for IL, but in order to accurately assess those problems, the degree to which the person is handicapped by those functional limitations in his vocational life, social life, familial life, and all other life roles n 1st be evaluated. Major problems may exist in one role, and only minor ones in another. For example, an individual might be able to work but be unable to live independently in his home and community. Since holding a job usually requires a person to move into the community, his problems with IL in the home could very well result in his being unable to accept employment that would otherwise be within his capability. Such complex problems as this are faced daily by those with severely handicapping conditions.

Both disabilities and their resulting handicaps are of increasing concern as one becomes older (Blake, 1981). Elderly people have disabilities more frequently than the general population, and therefore they are an important client group for IL services. It is important, then, that a definition of elderly be included in this discussion of terms.

ELDERLY

There is no clear answer to the question of who is elderly. Blake (1981) points out that most demographic studies use chronological age as a means of definition, choosing some arbitrary age, often 65, as the point at which people are described as elderly. The disadvantage of using chronological age as a guide, however, is that the problems associated with becoming old do not regularly occur with all people at some predetermined age.

Blake goes on to describe certain groups of people as perhaps becoming "old" earlier than others. He mentions that native Americans, as well as people who are developmentally disabled, have average life expectancies significantly lower than the total population. Does that mean that these groups become "old" at an earlier age? No one has yet answered that question, but certain problems associated with old age can certainly be found among those who are disabled at a younger chronological age. Recent follow-up studies of postpolio patients have uncovered certain problems that may indicate that old age arrives among people in this group as early as the midforties ("Are Polios Getting Older Faster?" 1981).

Therefore, in attempting to decide who is elderly it is important to focus upon functional problems rather than chronological age. For the purposes of this discussion, at least two factors can be mentioned that help to clarify the relationship of elderly people to ILR. First, "the age group for which disability is most common" is the older population (Blake, 1981, p. 26). The incidence of disability increases as people get older, especially after age 55. A result of this is that a large percentage of disabled people are middle-aged and older. Blake (1981) and Dunn (1981) indicate that two-thirds of all work-disabled persons are 40 years old or older. Older people, therefore, are of special interest in ILR because of their high incidence of disability and the associated high incidence of functional limitations.

Second, older people face the same social stigma, prejudice, and stereotyping that people who are disabled encounter (Benedict and Ganikos, 1981). These negative reactions and attitudes from society can greatly hinder the older person's effective performance in various life roles, and thus they represent real handicaps.

This combination of functional and social problems encountered by older people leads to a definition of elderly, emphasizing functional issues, that serves the purpose of this text. The term "elderly" refers to that point in life when the functional limitations that tend to be associated with advanced age present a significant handicap to the individual in relation to his or her desired roles in life. It is important to note that this definition of elderly is intended to identify those who would be served by ILR programs. Its emphasis upon functional limitations excludes older people who have experienced few problems in this regard. At the same time, it stresses that it is functional limitations rather than age alone that make older people an important client group for IL services.

At this point the reader should note a certain chain of thought regarding IL needs. First, one encounters people in society who are elderly, disabled, or both. Second, those people are handicapped in a variety of ways by the functional limitations resulting from their age or disability. The next link in this chain is the process through which these handicaps are overcome and the person's independence is restored. That process is commonly known as rehabilitation.

## REHABILITATION

The term "rehabilitation" has been defined as "the restoration of handicapped persons to the fullest physical, mental, social, vocational and economic usefulness of which they are capable" (International Labour Office, 1973, p. 1). This definition, or a variation of it, has been widely used for some time, but nevertheless it is somewhat misleading. It implies that rehabilitation is something done to, for, or on behalf of people who are handicapped. While that may be partly true, the definition fails to recognize the critically important role played by the handicapped person as the prime agent in the rehabilitation process. To develop a more adequate definition of rehabilitation, one should recognize that the handicapped person is the prime agent involved in a process that attacks the barriers imposed by a variety of handicapping factors interposed between the individual and his personal goals. Therefore, rehabilitation is defined as the process through which a handicapped individual eliminates, reduces, or circumvents the barriers that have limited or prevented his or her effective functioning.

To further clarify this definition of rehabilitation consider the example of Jason. Jason was recently rendered paraplegic by an accident on his job as a lineman for a utility company. Since he cannot continue his job, Jason would like to transfer into the drafting department, but several barriers have presented themselves. First, he obviously has a mobility impairment. He is using the services of a physical therapist to develop his upper body strength so that he will be able to maneuver himself about in a wheelchair. Since Jason lives alone, another major barrier for him is presented by the many activities of daily living that he routinely performed in the past but that now require some modifications on his part. For example, he will need to reorganize his kitchen so that he will be able to reach all the groceries, cooking utensils, and other items he will need, and he will need to learn to use his range, oven, washer, and dryer from his wheelchair. Jason plans to get help from an occupational therapist in a local IL center to help him learn to perform these tasks. Since transportation will also be a barrier, he plans to take a driver education course with hand controls installed on his car. Finally, Jason does not have the training required for a position as a draftsman in his company. To overcome that barrier he is making plans with a vocational rehabilitation counselor to enroll in a vocational-technical training program.

It is clear that a multitude of barriers are interposed between Jason and his goals of living independently and working as a draftsman. Jason's rehabilitation process is simply his effort to eliminate, reduce, or circumvent those barriers. His lack of training for the job he wants is a barrier that he can eliminate by going to school. He is reducing the barrier imposed by his impaired mobility by learning to use a wheelchair, and he will circumvent some of his problems with activities of daily living by learning new methods of achieving his objectives. In his rehabilitation process Jason will use the services of a physical therapist, an occupational therapist, a physician, a driving instructor, an educator, a rehabilitation counselor, and perhaps others as well. Each of these professionals will make an important contribution to Jason, but they will neither individually nor collectively "rehabilitate" him. They simply are participants in a multidisciplinary rehabilitation team of which Jason is both the central member and prime agent.

INDEPENDENT LIVING REHABILITATION (ILR)

Given the above broad definition of rehabilitation, one can define any specific type of rehabilitation by simply incorporating the barriers to be attacked in the rehabilitation process. For example, vocational rehabilitation is simply a rehabilitation process that addresses itself specifically to barriers that prevent the individual from working. ILR is then a rehabilitation process that addresses itself to the barriers preventing the individual from living as independently as he or she can and wants.

The concept of IL itself is a rather difficult term to describe. It is discussed in detail in Chapter 3. Parts 2 and 3 describe the wide range of services commonly used in the ILR process.

## HISTORICAL DEVELOPMENT
## OF THE INDEPENDENT LIVING CONCEPT

The concept of IL services has actually developed quite recently in this country. Some of the human service programs that make major contributions to the independence of people with severe disabilities, however, have existed for many years. To a large degree, the development of the IL concept has been both a cause and a result of the developments and progress made in these related programs. Therefore, to look at the historical development of the IL services concept is a rather complex task. It requires that one consider the development of a variety of human service programs and their contribution to IL, and it also requires that one appreciate the major role that severely disabled people have played in bringing about this new service concept.

Flynn and Nitsch (1980) have developed an "adoption of social innovations" framework that is helpful in understanding how social innovations such as IL services come to be accepted and implemented in society. Using that framework as a guide, the discussion that follows will attempt to clarify the historical development of independent living services.

The model of the adoption of social innovations (Figure 1.1) developed by Flynn and Nitsch (1980) is a two-phase, six-stage process with a "closed loop feedback structure" (p. 365). This model suggests that a given social innovation will first be adopted in theory (phase one), and that this theoretical adoption will occur in three stages: conceptualization, initial acceptance, and legislative legitimation. Adoption in practice (phase two) follows, and it also occurs in three stages: resource (re)allocation, widespread implementation, and societal institutionalization. Flynn and Nitsch describe this paradigm as follows:

> *Adoption-in-Theory.* During the conceptualization stage, the new idea or value system gradually evolves from some original insight into a well-articulated paradigm or model, and begins to be vigorously disseminated. Initial acceptance of the new paradigm is signaled by a period of limited, trial adoption by individuals and groups who are open to innovation and dissatisfied with the status quo. If the innovation gains the support of important segments of the target population, a period of legislative legitimation follows, during which appropriate legislation is enacted, regulations are issued, and judicial enforcement begins to occur.
>
> *Adoption-in-Practice.* At this point in the adoption process, the innovation faces a critical period of prolonged struggle against strong tendencies toward stable equilibrium and self-preservation by the old, entrenched value system. Bitter resistance is especially likely during the stage of resource (re)allocation, which signals the impending eclipse, in practice, of the old model. If sufficient resources are devoted to the new model, a stage of widespread implementation follows. Finally, the new way of thinking and acting must be protected against the constant threat of reversion by adequate measures of institutionalization. During this last stage, society as a whole moves from an attitude of external compliance or coercion to one of internalization, and creates safeguards to protect the integrity of the new paradigm. (P. 365)

ADOPTION-IN-PRACTICE | ADOPTION-IN-THEORY

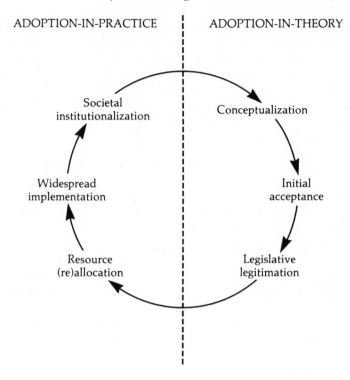

*Figure 1.1    Stages in the adoption cycle of a social innovation.*

## PHASE ONE: ADOPTION-IN-THEORY

The adoption-in-theory of IL as a human service goal is complete at this point. In view of the long history of services directed at the disabled in this country, the idea of IL took a long time to appear. Yet after IL first became a topic of public debate around 1970, it quickly became a popular cause and found its way into major legislation by 1978. The conceptualization, initial acceptance, and legislative legitimation of the IL concept will be discussed in detail below.

**Stage One: Conceptualization**    In considering the conceptualization of IL services one might consider the concept of personal independence that was discussed in the introduction to this chapter. That concept suggests that maximum personal independence has been a matter of importance in this country since it was founded and even before. If that is true, then why is it that personal independence for people who are disabled has only recently been a widespread concern? Perhaps part of the answer lies in the complex set of historical roots that created in this society an extremely pervasive work ethic, which has tended to guide human service organizations toward occupationally oriented service efforts and, at the same time, has tended to discredit anyone who does not or cannot work. As a result, there has been a heavy emphasis upon vocational service agencies for disabled people, and little effort has been given to other matters.

To illustrate this historical trend, consider the reaction of this society to disabled people during its early history. During the early colonial era, people who would be dependent on a community because of advanced age, ill health, or disability were commonly excluded from immigration rights by colonial legislation (Lenihan, 1977). The reason for this was that these people were considered to be burdens (that is, they could not work and perhaps required care from others) that the community could not afford. As the colonies became more economically able, they began to offer aid to persons in need through various types of almshouses, which provided room, board, and varying degrees of care to those who were disabled, sick, old, poor, or dependent for some other reason. Unfortunately, the people in these almshouses were usually seen as pitiful victims, and there was virtually no hope that they could ever join the mainstream of society as equal citizens.

The importance of the work ethic in early America in influencing services to disabled persons can be seen in laws governing the Northwest Territory. Lenihan (1977) quotes laws requiring each town overseer to "assess taxes on the town inhabitants to provide 'houses and places, and a convenient stock of hemp, flax, thread and other ware and stuff, for setting to work such persons, as apply for relief, and are capable of working; and also for relieving such poor, old, blind, impotent, and lame persons, or other persons not able to work, within the said townships, respectively; who shall therewith be maintained and provided for' " (pp. 16–17). A trend was being started even then of providing work as a means of relief for those who needed help and who could work. Unfortunately, this trend also involved such negative features as choosing for the needy person the type of work he or she would be engaged in and having that work available in a special place apart from the rest of society.

Less than a half-century later, Samuel Gridley Howe began his work in Boston with blind and retarded people. Howe introduced ideas much like those in vogue today. He believed that blind children should receive education individualized to meet their needs and that they should be trained for jobs available in their communities (Lenihan, 1977). Unfortunately these noble aspirations were never realized, except in the work of Howe and some of his students. The prevailing attitudes in society would not let Howe's innovative recommendations become reality, and as Ferleger and Boyd (1980) point out, the model educational and job-training programs he envisioned deteriorated to the life-strangling institutions of the mid-1900s.

The emphasis on work-oriented programs is also evident in the private charitable organizations of the nineteenth century. Rubin and Roessler (1978) point out that such organizations were becoming widespread during the latter half of the nineteenth century and that their prevailing attitude was that "giving anyone anything that they could earn via their own labors was to reduce their incentive to work and contribute to their moral deterioration" (p. 15). Thus, any assistance provided to persons in need was likely to be heavily directed toward a work goal.

These examples from pre-twentieth-century America illustrate how important the work ethic has been in influencing services to the disabled. Nineteenth-century service efforts either attempted to provide work for the disabled individual or isolated the person from society in some type of almshouse facility. Neither type of assistance recognized the legitimacy of personal independence for people so severely disabled that they could not work. With the arrival of the twentieth century, service programs for disabled people grew in number and in their capacity to help, but they changed little in their basic work-oriented approaches.

Among the earliest developments in the twentieth century was the enactment of workers' compensation laws. As this society became industrialized, the incidence of occupational injuries increased significantly. As a result, many people incurred high medical expenses and, at the same time, lost their ability to work and earn an income. These people were quickly impoverished and had little assistance on which they could depend. In 1908 the federal government enacted a workers' compensation law for federal employees (Bitter, 1979), and in 1910 New York became the first state to pass complete workers' compensation legislation (Rubin and Roessler, 1978). This new response to industrial accidents spread quickly, and by 1921 forty-five of the states and territories had legislated some type of workers' compensation protection (Obermann, 1965; Rubin and Roessler, 1978). Workers' compensation programs provided critically important income protection for people injured on the job, but they obviously were not at all concerned with the nonworking disabled person.

Vocational rehabilitation programs were the other major governmental response to disability in the early twentieth century. During and after World War I there was great sympathy in this country for soldiers who had become disabled during the war. The United States had paid pensions and other compensation to soldiers injured in military service previously, but World War I veterans received a new type of benefit. Through the Soldier Rehabilitation (Smith-Sears) Act of 1918, Congress authorized the provision of vocational rehabilitation services to disabled veterans. These services were designed to fit the veteran, primarily through education and training, for a new occupation (Obermann, 1965; Rubin and Roessler, 1978). As one might expect, the provision of vocational rehabilitation services for disabled veterans soon led to the belief that these services would be beneficial for all citizens, and efforts were quickly underway to obtain vocational rehabilitation services for civilians. These efforts resulted in the Vocational Rehabilitation Act of 1920, which provided services for civilians much like those available to veterans.

The emergence of vocational rehabilitation programs was perhaps the most important early development relative to IL programs. Vocational rehabilitation programs have been the major service delivery system for disabled people in the United States. Much of the technological progress that has increased the ability of a severely disabled person to live independently has been supported by vocational rehabilitation programs. Much of the leadership in bringing into existence current IL programs has come from people involved in vocational rehabilitation. Yet, ironically, the emphasis upon the "vocational" in vocational rehabilitation has perhaps delayed the full conceptualization and eventual implementation of IL programs.

The early vocational rehabilitation programs implemented as a result of the 1920 law were designed primarily to provide vocational training for physically disabled people (Rubin and Roessler, 1978). The mentally disabled were not included, and in fact very few people with severe disabilities were served by these early programs. The situation improved somewhat in 1943, when Congress passed the Barden-LaFollette Act, which included people who were mentally ill or mentally retarded as legitimate recipients of vocational rehabilitation services. Support for programs designed to serve the blind was also authorized. In addition to expanding the clientele served by state vocational rehabilitation agencies, the law expanded the services that could be provided to include medical services (physical restoration) and maintenance for people involved in a vocational rehabilitation program (Rubin and Roessler, 1978).

Up until the 1960s, the number of services offered by vocational rehabilitation programs continued to grow, but the vocational emphasis was maintained. Verville (1979) points out that during this period all nonvocational rehabilitation programs were excluded from consideration by Congress and by rehabilitation leaders themselves. One result of this emphasis was that vocational rehabilitation, even though it had been a major government program with a proven record of successful performance, was not the vehicle chosen for implementing expanded social services to a variety of people in need during the 1960s. For example, the Mental Retardation Facilities and Community Mental Health Centers Construction Act of 1963 offered expanded services to mentally retarded citizens. Yet, since nonvocational goals were to be emphasized, these services were not directed through the vocational rehabilitation program (Verville, 1979).

In the late 1960s and early 1970s, some vocational rehabilitation leaders advocated a broader nonvocational role for rehabilitation programs. However, legislation passed by Congress in 1972 that would have begun to move rehabilitation in that direction was vetoed by President Nixon. The reason for the veto was that the legislation "strayed too far from the essential vocational objective of the program" (Verville, 1979, p. 448).

Thus, the vocational rehabilitation program, which was responsible for much aid to disabled people who could go to work as a result of receiving services, was not able to assist the nonvocationally able disabled person at all. Indeed, the resistance of Congress and of rehabilitation professionals to nonvocational efforts may have been responsible for much delay in the development of programs such as IL.

The physically and mentally disabled people, many of them severely disabled, whose needs were not being met by governmental vocational rehabilitation programs, made their needs and desires known in the early 1970s more than ever before. Many began to take action that would soon culminate in the clear conceptualization of ILR service programs. These actions included testifying before congressional committees regarding the real needs of severely disabled individuals and developing consumer initiated and managed IL programs around the nation (Verville, 1979). The importance of these consumer efforts was further emphasized in the formation of the American Coalition of Citizens with Disabilities (ACCD), and in the White House Conference on Handicapped Individuals, a result of the 1974 Rehabilitation Act Amendments. The consumer movement, begun during the early 1970s, was concerned with needs reaching far beyond vocational services. The aggressive actions of severely disabled individuals were triggered in part by the failure of the traditional vocational rehabilitation program to respond to their most pressing needs. Thus, the conceptualization of IL programs has been partly a result of consumer reaction to the inadequacies of the vocational rehabilitation program.

Another trend in the early 1970s also contributed to the conceptualization of IL programs. For the mentally disabled person, the "normalization" principle as espoused by Wolfensberger (1980) has meant the development of major new service program designs. The trend in services for the mentally disabled in this decade has been captured by terms such as "mainstreaming" and "deinstitutionalization." The mentally disabled are being assisted in moving out of abnormal institutional environments and into more normal community settings. A major part of the new service paradigm involved in normalization is providing IL services for the disabled person.

**Stage Two: Initial Acceptance**   The initial acceptance of a new service model is signaled by its adoption on a trial basis. Usually such adoption is by groups interested in changing the status quo (Flynn and Nitsch, 1980).

The initial acceptance of IL service models was intertwined with consumer efforts to introduce innovative service concepts. In the early 1970s, successful IL programs were developed, primarily by consumer-oriented groups. These early programs were developed independently, but they shared many basic ideas, such as consumer management, serving as advocates for severely disabled people in the community, and assisting each individual to define his or her own goals of independence. They set patterns that later, more extensive efforts at ILR would follow. Among the notable early programs were the Berkeley Center for Independent Living, the Boston Center for Independent Living, and the New Options program in Houston. The current ILR movement owes much to the creative leadership of those involved in developing these innovative programs.

**Stage Three: Legislative Legitimation**   IL programs finally achieved legislative legitimacy in the Rehabilitation, Comprehensive Services, and Developmental Disabilities Legislation of 1978, Public Law 95-602, often referred to as the Rehabilitation Amendments of 1978. Specifically, it is Title VII of this legislation, entitled "Comprehensive Services for Independent Living," that provides this legislative base.

The services authorized in Title VII are divided into four parts, only one of which was initially funded by Congress. Part A, entitled "Comprehensive Services," was one of the three parts that were not initially funded. This part would, if funded, allow state vocational rehabilitation agencies to provide "any appropriate vocational rehabilitation service . . . and any other service that will enhance the ability of a handicapped individual to live independently and function within his family and community and, if appropriate, secure and maintain appropriate employment" (Public Law 95-602). This is the part of the law that would have the greatest effect on the largest number of severely disabled people if it were funded and implemented. It would allow each state's vocational rehabilitation agency to make IL services available to all its citizens in need of and eligible for such services. This part of the law would also authorize the provision of some services, such as housing modifications, and necessary adaptive and assistive devices and equipment, which are not authorized in other parts of the law.

Part B of Title VII, entitled "Centers for Independent Living," was funded by Congress, and it has supported the initial implementation of federally sponsored IL service programs throughout the country. Part B provides for "the establishment and operation of independent living centers" that can provide a wide range of services designed to enhance the ability of a severely disabled individual to live independently. This part of the law is not as extensive in scope as Part A, nor will the centers funded by it be able to serve all regions of each state, as the programs authorized in Part A would be able to do. This part of the Rehabilitation Amendments of 1978, however, has certainly made a historic contribution to the IL movement in this country, simply because funds made available through it have enabled every state to begin offering some type of IL services.

Part C of Title VII, entitled "Independent Living Services for Older Blind Individuals" and Part D, entitled "General Provisions," were the other parts of the law that were not initially funded. These parts would, if funded, provide services "designed to assist an older blind individual to adjust to his blindness by becoming more able to care for his individual needs" and would provide protection and advocacy services for severely handicapped individuals (Public Law 95-602).

All four parts of Title VII include provisions to ensure that the disabled consumers have some input in the programs it authorizes. One of these important provisions is that each client will have an individualized IL program (ILP) written specifically for him or her. This ILP is to be developed jointly by the IL center's staff representative and the client, the client's parent or guardian, or the client's representative.

At the time of this writing, the implementation of the IL provisions of Public Law 95-602 is in its infancy. It is too early to judge the effectiveness of these infant programs, but it is encouraging to note that efforts to implement them are widespread.

There have been other important legislative contributions in support of IL. As is obvious throughout this text, successful IL programs require the services and resources of a wide variety of human service programs. The more important programs are briefly summarized here.

First, the Rehabilitation Act of 1973 was one of the most important pieces of legislation for severely disabled people in this country's history, and without it IL programs would face much more severe challenges than they do. In a sense the Rehabilitation Act of 1973 can be considered the "trailblazer" for the IL provisions in the 1978 Amendments. It has been mentioned earlier that proposed rehabilitation legislation in 1972 was vetoed by President Nixon. That legislation had provisions for IL services. But even though the legislation was vetoed, it became evident that Congress was ready to recognize a new role for rehabilitation. In the subsequent 1973 legislation, Congress omitted the word "vocational" from rehabilitation legislation for the first time in the 53-year history of such programs. The 1973 law also required that state rehabilitation agencies give priority of services to severely disabled clients, and that clients be actively involved in their own rehabilitation planning and decision making. These provisions began a trend of moving the objective of rehabilitation programs beyond a purely vocational role and toward serving severely disabled people.

The most important effect of the Rehabilitation Act of 1973 comes from the strong support it gives to basic rights for disabled people. DeLoach and Greer (1981) provide an excellent discussion of legislation affecting disabled people, and they state that one of the three most important contributions of the 1973 law is "its establishment of a civil rights provision for the handicapped" (p. 148). This provision is found in Section 504 of the law, which states, "No otherwise qualified handicapped individual in the United States . . . shall, solely by reason of his handicap, be excluded from the participation in, be denied the benefits of, or be subjected to discrimination under any program or activity receiving Federal financial assistance" (Public Law 93-112). That simple statement has had tremendous impact on this society in opening doors (literally) to disabled people that had never before been open. The current IL movement would be severely handicapped itself were it not for Section 504 requirements that programs receiving federal financial assistance make themselves available to disabled persons. Curb cuts in sidewalks, specially designated handicapped parking spaces, accessible public transportation, ramps into public buildings, universities with special services for disabled students, equal employment practices, and many other changes that one can see throughout this society are either partially or wholly a result of Section 504. Thus, its importance as a prerequisite to successful IL programs is obvious. Without it society would be so restrictive that services designed to increase personal independence would be futile.

In addition to the 1973 Rehabilitation Act, several other laws and human service programs are important in establishing the legislative authority for important components of IL service programs. These important supportive programs and laws are briefly mentioned below. They each play an important part in a complex IL service delivery system, which is described in detail in Chapter 9.

The *Housing and Community Development Act* provides housing assistance to disabled and elderly persons. It also helps ensure the availablity of housing accessible to people with physical impairments (DeLoach and Greer, 1981). The *Social Security Act* of 1935 and its amendments in 1954 and 1965 provide income protection for those who retire at age 62 or 65 and for those who become disabled before retirement age (Rubin and Roessler, 1978). *Supplemental Security Income* (SSI) is "designed to assist the aged, blind, and disabled who have limited income and little or no other resources" (Gives, 1978, p. 186). SSI is primarily an income supplement program, as its name implies. *Medicare* is available to provide medical services to those over 65 who are receiving Social Security benefits, or to those who have received Social Security Disability Insurance (SSDI) benefits for two consecutive years or more, or to those "who need dialysis treatment or a kidney transplant" and are receiving SSDI (Gives, 1978, p. 189). *Medicaid* is the term often used to designate the individual states' assistance to low-income people who need medical care but do not qualify for Medicare. Services available under state Medicaid programs obviously vary more than do Medicare services (Gives, 1978). The *Comprehensive Older Americans Act Amendments* provide for a variety of social services to homebound disabled and elderly people (DeLoach and Greer, 1981).

It would be naive to attribute the legislative legitimation of IL services solely to the Rehabilitation Amendments of 1978. No other area of human service needs has as many important contributing services as IL has. All of the many programs and laws mentioned above have been important in establishing the legislative base necessary to support comprehensive IL service programs.

## PHASE TWO: ADOPTION-IN-PRACTICE

At the time of this writing, the IL services concept is probably best characterized as being at the balance point between adoption-in-theory and adoption-in-practice. Flynn and Nitsch (1980) point out that innovative service delivery concepts will face tough opposition at the point of adoption-in-practice, and that certainly is the case with the fledgling IL service programs now in existence. The stages of resource (re)allocation, widespread implementation, and institutionalization are discussed below.

**Stage Four: Resource (Re)allocation**   An innovative service delivery system is likely to face its greatest resistance at the point where resource (re)allocation is required. When the time comes to invest money in a new program, the real commitment of society to that new program is tested, and is often found lacking. This is the test now facing IL programs.

It is an unfortunate circumstance, purely accidental and beyond anyone's control, that new IL service programs are trying to solidly establish their funding resources at a time when this society is cutting back on almost all social programs. As a result, the resistance to full implementation and adequate funding of these programs is greater than one would normally expect to find. For example, the IL program established in the author's own community was originally funded from a three-year grant authorized in the 1978 Rehabilitation Amendments. This grant was in the amount of $200,000 for the first year of operation, with the amount to be decreased in each succeeding year, and finally with all federal support to be withdrawn after the third year. The pressure on the staff in such a program is obvious and intense. They must somehow find other sources of funding or else find their program extinct before it ever has a chance to prove itself.

The final solution to the problem of funding IL programs will likely involve both economic and humanitarian concerns. It is important that IL programs quickly demonstrate that they offer an effective service delivery system that, in the most cost-effective way, significantly helps clients to achieve higher levels of independence. A more detailed discussion of this issue is found in Chapter 4.

**Stage Five: Widespread Implementation**   At the time of this writing, IL service programs have achieved widespread implementation in a rather tenuous sense. Some of the older programs, such as the Berkeley Center for Independent Living in Berkeley, California, and Paraquad in Saint Louis, Missouri, have been in existence long enough to demonstrate their ability to survive even in adverse economic conditions, but the many new programs that have been implemented since the 1978 Rehabilitation Amendments have not proven their viability over time. These fledgling programs are struggling to establish themselves in a very difficult economic climate. Unfortunately, only time will reveal whether or not they will survive, an event that depends to a large degree on the effectiveness of the programs, on the political pressures of disabled consumers and advocates, and on economic circumstances beyond the control of either disabled people or the professional staff of IL programs.

**Stage Six: Societal Institutionalization**   If IL programs are able to establish solid financial support and prove themselves as effective service delivery systems, then their effectiveness and existence must continue to be protected through societal institutionalization. This is the process of society adopting the new service model completely as its own. In the words of Flynn and Nitsch (1980) "society must internalize and safeguard it against the forces of lowered expectancies and performance decay that seem to be intrinsic to all social systems" (p. 387). These authors go on to suggest that voluntary associations, consumer advocacy groups, and effective program evaluation can all contribute to societal institutionalization.

One of the most exciting aspects of being involved in the development of IL programs is that those involved now have the opportunity to improve on the older human service models. These new programs have the chance to avoid the mistakes built into the older models and at the same time to incorporate better program evaluation, more cooperation with voluntary associations and consumer groups, and other measures that will help to maintain high quality programs.

It is important that this opportunity for improved program design not be missed, because mistakes made now and incorporated into the way these service programs function will cause problems for many years to come. In fact, programs that do not function at their maximum effectiveness may become institutionalized just as well as programs that do. When this occurs, unfortunately, the clients of these programs bear the consequences. As discussed earlier the vocational rehabilitation program for its first 58 years of existence did not serve clients who did not have a vocational goal, no matter how severe their needs may have been. The policy that this government program was to be strictly vocational in nature was protected by the forces of societal institutionalization, even though the need for change was obvious to many severely disabled people.

Katz and Kahn (1978) discuss this tendency of organizations to protect and maintain themselves without loss of system character, and they claim that a common side effect of this phenomenon is that system character is not only maintained but intensified. They refer to this as "system dynamics" (pp. 47–48). Furthermore, they state that "both the major system and the component subsystems are characterized by their own dynamic or complex of motivational forces that move a given structure toward becoming more like what it basically is. For example, a hospital for mental patients organized as a custodial institution tends over time to become more of a custodial institution unless it is subject to new inputs from its supporting environment . . ." (p. 48). Thus vocational rehabilitation agencies understandably tended not only to resist changes of their vocational nature but even to intensify that nature. Input from the supporting environment (in this case, disabled consumers) was not only desirable but absolutely necessary in order to make basic changes.

The point of this discussion for the staff of newly established IL programs is that they should take care in moving their programs toward the point of achieving societal institutionalization. They will want to design their programs in such a manner that they will be happy with the essential nature of the programs over time, because that nature is likely to be maintained and even intensified. More importantly, they should also design their programs to receive maximum input from the supporting environment. This can be done, as Flynn and Nitsch suggest, by involving consumer groups and voluntary associations and by quality program evaluation. This type of continued input from external sources is the best assurance of protecting service quality over long periods of time.

## SUMMARY

This chapter has presented and defined the most basic terms used throughout this text. The evolution of IL as a human services goal has been discussed in terms of Flynn and Nitsch's model of social innovations adoption. The adoption-in-theory of IL services was completed with the passage of the 1978 Rehabilitation Amendments. The IL programs authorized by this legislation provide the unifying structure necessary to make the ILR service delivery system in this country an effective means of helping severely disabled people to achieve the personal independence they desire. Critical tests still lie ahead, however, as rehabilitation professionals and disabled consumers attempt to bring these new IL programs to the point of full adoption-in-practice. The remainder of this text will discuss how the goal of IL can be further clarified and justified, how necessary support services can be obtained and used, what types of IL programs are available, and what factors determine success in IL. It is hoped that these discussions will enable the reader to understand what IL programs are supposed to accomplish, to evaluate their actual performance, and perhaps to contribute to their eventual success.

# 2

## A Case for Coordinating Independent Living Services for People of All Ages

Johnny D., an athletic 19-year-old, is recovering from an accident that crushed his spine at the level of the sixth cervical vertebra (C6). His physician informs Johnny's parents that, with rehabilitation, Johnny will be independent in his self-care, will be able to drive his own modified vehicle, and will have the stamina to work at a wide range of jobs for which he is qualified, despite the limitations imposed by his quadriplegia.

Richard M., in a different medical setting in a different section of the country, is also 19, of similar intelligence, and has the same high degree of self-discipline and motivation as Johnny. Richard also shares Johnny's physical limitations, since his cord, too, was severed at the level of the sixth cervical vertebra. His physician, however, informs Richard's parents that their son, while able to feed himself and push his wheelchair for short distances on smooth, level surfaces, will require attendant care for the rest of his life to help him bathe, dress, transfer to and from his wheelchair, and attend to his toileting needs.

27

Which physician is correct in his prognosis? A problem of rehabilitation is that, even when the factors of age, body weight, general physical health, intelligence and degree of motivation are held constant, there can be varying, often contradictory, results. In the cases of Johnny and Richard, both physicians could be correct (Bitter, 1979; Hylbert and Hylbert, 1979; Trigiano and Mitchell, 1970).

Prognoses like Johnny's can be fulfilled when comprehensive rehabilitation services are available: skilled medical care, dedicated rehabilitation professionals experienced in working with spinal cord injuries, adaptive aids, modifications in the home and community, and, finally, a variety of support services that can be utilized when needed. Today, Johnny's prognosis is typical of that given to people with this type and degree of disability in such outstanding rehabilitation centers as Craig Rehabilitation Hospital in Englewood, Colorado, or the Texas Institute of Rehabilitation and Research (TIRR) in Houston.

Yet hundreds of Richards are disabled every year in automobile and sports accidents and do not receive the comprehensive services they require. Unlike Johnny, they live out their lives more physically, economically, and socially restricted than their disabilities warrant. They may be served by professionals who are overworked or whose training and expectations reflect the now-outdated rehabilitation realities of the early 1970s or before. In some cases, these Richards are not able to afford the requisite adaptive aids and are not otherwise provided with them (Bruck, 1978). They may live in communities that are unresponsive to or incapable of responding to the needs of severely disabled residents. And what is true for the 10,000 to 12,000 young adults who acquire spinal cord injuries every year in the United States (Goldenson, Dunham, and Dunham, 1978; Lancaster, 1976) is also true for the mentally retarded, those born with physical defects, and those who acquire other types of physically disabling conditions.

Independent living as a service paradigm (see Chapter 1) is designed to eliminate inconsistent rehabilitation outcomes. Independent living theory, fully translated into prescribed rehabilitation services, would mean that physicians like Johnny's would usually be correct, and physicians like Richard's would change their expectations or be phased out of rehabilitation services. A well-established, widely supported independent living basis for all rehabilitation-related services could benefit not only the approximately 36 million disabled children and adults in our society, but the rest of society as well. Societal benefits would accrue, first, from the salvaging of the too-often neglected human resource that disabled people represent and, second, from the reduction in the costs of maintaining disabled people within society without providing them with the services that would allow them to be contributing citizens (see Chapter 4).

This chapter will

1. describe the evolution of service delivery formats designed to promote independent living,

2. describe the general goals of independent living,

3. explain why independent living (IL) services are designed to be available to disabled people on a life-long basis,

4. relate the philosophy of normalization to the philosophy of independent living,

5. describe the three levels of independent functioning,

6. explain why IL goals are best determined by client need rather than by age or disability type.

## THE EVOLUTION OF INDEPENDENT LIVING PROGRAM MODELS

Although the concept of independent living goes back to the first civilian rehabilitation act, the Smith-Fess Act of 1920, which included homemaking as a feasible vocational objective, the first definitive IL program began operating in the late 1940s. This early prototype of today's IL programs was the system of services offered to disabled University of Illinois students through the university's Division of Rehabilitation-Education Services.

### PHASE ONE: THE ILLINOIS MODEL

In 1948 the University of Illinois began offering a program of special supportive services to severely disabled veterans of World War II. It soon expanded its program to include disabled civilians as well. The Illinois model incorporated many of the categories of service offered by IL programs established through the 1978 Amendments but differed significantly in its procedures for establishing eligibility and in its concept of independent living. Among the services routinely offered students were accessible undergraduate, graduate, and married student housing; wheelchair accessible transportation; specialized medical care; educational support services; peer counseling; development and repair of assistive devices; and training in the activities of daily living (ADL), including dressing, bathing, toileting, housekeeping and driving skills.

**Selection Criteria**   Prior to the 1973 Rehabilitation Act, which made it illegal for universities receiving government funds to discriminate on the basis of handicap, the Illinois program screened disabled applicants for admission to the university on the basis of whether or not their disabilities were severe enough to prevent them from living in university dormitories without assistance. When disabled people applied for admittance, their applications were channeled directly to the Division of Rehabilitation-Education Services. Then a personal interview was scheduled, during which the division's staff made a determination of how physically independent each applicant was. Those who were self-sufficient and who met the university's general requirements for admittance were admitted. Those who were judged to have no potential for coping with the demands of daily living without assistance were denied admittance. Those who were not self-sufficient at the time of the interview but who were thought capable of functioning without assistance were admitted provisionally, with the understanding that they would undergo intensive training in self-care skills the week prior to student orientation week. At the conclusion of the week of functional training, applicants who were functioning independently were accepted into the university and applicants who still required assistance were not.

**Definition of Independence**   According to the Illinois model, independence is defined as the physical ability to live without assistance. Even today, although the law prohibits the university from denying admittance to those who require assistance in their ADL, undergraduate or unmarried students who require attendant care live in the Beckwith Living Center, a specially designed housing unit on the university's campus. The continuing emphasis of the Illinois model on physical independence is illustrated by a quote from the Division's brochure on the Beckwith Center: "individual instruction and training are offered in those skills that enable the student to assume greater responsibility for self and to lessen dependence on others. Experience suggests that many can achieve complete or near complete independence levels, each in his or her own way."

PHASE TWO: THE GRASS-ROOTS MODEL

In the early 1970s, prior to the passage of the 1978 Amendments, numerous grass-roots IL centers and programs were established. Many of them failed, but many continue to serve disabled people today (Laurie, 1977). Some of these centers and programs, like the

Berkeley Center for Independent Living (CIL) in California, were initiated, staffed and operated primarily by physically disabled persons. Others, like Timbers in Wichita, Kansas, were initiated and operated by church groups or organizations such as United Cerebral Palsy (Laurie, 1977).

These grass-roots programs differ from the Illinois program in several ways: program recipients do not have to be college students; there tends to be greater consumer input and control; and independence is a relative concept in which the ability to control one's life is emphasized as much as the ability to exercise some degree of physical self-sufficiency. Because of the number of grass-roots programs, each operating independently, there is a greater diversity among them than among programs that have been established under the federal guidelines for Part B of the 1978 Amendments.

## PHASE THREE: COMPREHENSIVE INDEPENDENT LIVING PROGRAMS

The passage of the 1978 Amendments legitimized through federal legislation the provision of IL services as a social service paradigm. Although programs established through Title VII of the 1978 Amendments were implemented through the existing vocational rehabilitation bureaucracy, people who previously might have been denied services that were vocational in intent became eligible for IL services. According to the eligibility criterion established by the Amendments:

> Services may be provided under this title to any individual whose ability to engage or continue in employment, or whose ability to function independently in his family or community, is so limited by the severity of his disability that Vocational or Comprehensive Rehabilitation Services appreciably more costly and of appreciably greater duration than those Vocational or Comprehensive Rehabilitation Services required for the rehabilitation of a handicapped individual are required to improve significantly either his ability to engage in employment or his ability to function independently in his family or community. Priority of services under this part shall be given to individuals not served by other provisions of the Act. (Public Law 95-602)

## WHAT IS INDEPENDENT LIVING?

Under the Illinois model, independent living services were considered those services that, if successful, result in disabled people living totally self-sufficient lives, freed from the need to rely on others for their self-care needs. Although under the Illinois model many severely physically disabled individuals attained a degree of physical self-sufficiency that exceeded the expectations of specialists in rehabilitation medicine (Trigiano and Mitchell, 1970), being human, they never attained a state of total self-sufficiency. Independent living services are not designed to transform people with varying types and degrees of disability into superhuman beings, for even those who are not disabled are not totally self-sufficient in our highly specialized, interdependent society. Independent living services are, however, intended to enhance one's self-sufficiency to the greatest degree possible, considering one's physical, emotional, and social circumstances.

Neither is independent living a static state of being. It is inaccurate to assume that once IL services have proven successful, that once an assessment of a person's competencies and limitations has been made and appropriate measures have been taken to enhance those competencies and minimize those limitations, no further services should be required. Such an assumption fails to take into account detrimental changes in health or living situations that may occur more frequently in people with certain disabling conditions. For example, when people disabled from polio reach their forties and fifties, they often experience a sudden and, as yet, unexplained loss of muscle strength. The resulting decrease in their respiratory ability, along with an accelerated degeneration of the motor neurons in their peripheral nervous systems, creates a need for further rehabilitation services for them, in their lifestyles, in the assistive devices they use, and in the avocational and vocational activities they pursue (Laurie, 1980, 1981).

In the main, especially in programs established under the 1978 Amendments, IL services should be designed to help disabled people of all ages function as independently and in as consistent a manner as possible, regardless of changes in their physical states or social environments. Especially for those with severe physical disabilities, a thin line exists between independence and total dependence. For many, independence or dependence is always a matter of degree and the degree of independence or dependence experienced often rests on factors external to the individual. In northern areas of the country, for example, an employed person with a mobility impairment may have no difficulty driving to and from work in the spring, summer, and fall. But when ice or snow accumulates on sidewalks, driveways, and roads, the person who required no assistance in clement weather may require a great deal of help to move easily and safely over the walkways and driveways at his or her home and job site.

## INDEPENDENT LIVING SERVICES
## FOR OLDER DISABLED PEOPLE

In 1978 twenty-two percent of those over 45 years of age who were accepted for vocational rehabilitation services were rehabilitated (Blake, 1981). Traditionally, older physically disabled people have been significantly underrepresented among those served by existing vocational rehabilitation programs. Under early rehabilitation legislation it was assumed that older and elderly disabled people were underserved because they had little or no vocational potential. The 1978 Amendments, however, provide for services to people who do not have the potential to become gainfully employed. In fact, as Williams (1981) points out, the last sentence of the section dealing with the criteria for eligibility, namely, "Priority of services under this part shall be given to individuals not served by other provisions of the Act," indicates that older disabled people are among those who should be given priority in receiving IL services.

Nevertheless older disabled people continue to be underserved by IL programs established under the 1978 Amendments. Of the five demonstration projects funded by the Rehabilitation Services Administration (RSA) in 1978, only one mentions older disabled people as part of their designated target population. Among the IL programs surveyed by the Independent Living Research Utilization Project, none specifies older disabled people in its description of the categories it serves (ILRUP, 1979).

Two factors appear to contribute to the lack of IL services specifically designed to meet the needs of elderly disabled people. First, "physically disabled person" is synonymous in many service providers' minds with "young physically disabled person." Therefore, "the physically disabled" are viewed as being concerned with employment, marriage, raising their families, establishing a home, and so on. Second, the consumers involved in the founding and operation of both the grass-roots programs and the federally sponsored programs tend to be young, active, physically disabled people. There has been resentment on the part of young disabled people toward federal policies that group services and programs for them with programs and services designed for elderly people who may or may not be disabled. For example, public housing for the elderly incorporates wheelchair accessible units that are available both to young disabled adults and to elderly disabled people, but accessible public housing is not made available that is strictly for younger persons. The result appears to be an age bias on the part of many consumers who are engaged in the policy-setting aspects of recently established IL programs.

The lack of IL services for older disabled people, for whatever reason, is unfortunate because disabled people over 45 have as great a need for these services as do those from 16 to 45 years of age (Benedict and Ganikos, 1981; Blake, 1981; Bozarth, 1981; Williams, 1981). For example, veterans disabled in World War II and in Korea, if they had families, are already grandparents and, if they were employed, are retired or thinking about retirement. Although they may not share the exact living concerns of those who are establishing homes, families and careers, they do as a group, according to Williams (1981), require the same types of IL services as other disabled people, such as mobility assistance, homemaker services and attendant care, and information and referral services. Moreover, shifting social demographics emphasize the need for addressing the IL needs, especially, of the elderly physically disabled. According to the Urban Institute, in 1977 of the 10 million noninstitutionalized severely disabled people in the United States, "4,000,000, or 40 percent, were 65 or older." By 1984, the Institute estimated, there would be 13 million severely disabled people and "5.5 million, or more than one-third, of those 13 million persons will be 65 or older" (Blake, 1981; Williams, 1981).

## GOALS OF INDEPENDENT LIVING SERVICES

To enable severely disabled people of all ages to function to their maximum potential, four general objectives for IL services have been identified. These four goals are

1. to help disabled persons live as independently as possible,
2. to maintain their highest level of functional independence as long as possible,
3. to live as fully integrated into the community as possible, and
4. to live each day in the same manner as nondisabled persons of the same age and background as far as possible.

### ATTAINING OPTIMUM INDEPENDENCE

**Establishing Client Goals** Before formulating a client's IL program, the IL counselor, in conjunction with the client, must decide which behaviors would constitute optimum independent function for the client in question. In reaching a viable decision, two questions should be considered: (1) what level of independent function is possible for the client, and (2) what level of independent functioning is feasible for the client? For example, a client might be physically able to stop using a wheelchair for mobility and start using braces and crutches, but in doing so might expend so much time and energy that, overall, he would be functioning at a lower level of independence in other areas of his life than before.

The key to effective IL services is setting objectives that fulfill an individual's potential without creating excessive physiological and psychological stress. In the Illinois model, the decision on how independently a person could function was based on the experience of program staff with similarly disabled individuals. In the grass-roots model and in programs established through RSA, disabled individuals play a major role in the decision-making process.

Client participation can be implemented in one of several ways. At Rancho de los Amigos in Downy, California, IL objectives are determined in a five-step process. First, the referring counselor lists the ADL skills he or she believes the client can master. Second, the client describes the activities he or she regularly carries out successfully. Third, the client describes the level of independence in ADL he or she believes is possible after appropriate services have been received. Fourth, the client is provided with the designated training and assistive devices. Fifth, the client's success in achieving the IL objectives is evaluated and, if necessary, the last three steps are repeated.

In order to establish objectives that are appropriate for each individual receiving IL services, it is necessary to take into account the lifestyle of the average person in the subsociety to which that individual belongs. To achieve acceptance and integration, disabled people must attain, or closely approximate, certain socially sanctioned goals that signify responsible adulthood in our society: economic independence, emotional independence, and marriage (Wright, 1960). Or, inasmuch as optimum psychological and social adjustment must be considered in the context of a society's basic values, the IL paradigm must reflect the social values of the 1980s, in which a lasting, mutually satisfying, intimate relationship may serve as a socially sanctioned substitute for marriage. In addition, the IL paradigm must include a fourth element that is assumed for adults who are not disabled—independence in basic self-care and homemaking activities (DeLoach and Greer, 1981).

Therefore, those who offer services that are intended to enhance the independence of the disabled must take into account all the essentials of a so-called normal lifestyle and then interpret these essentials in terms of behaviors that are within their capabilities and are supported through social resources. For disabled people, financial self-sufficiency may be attained through remunerative employment or some state, federal, or private income maintenance program. Emotional self-sufficiency may be defined as having confidence in one's ability and having the motivation to lead a self-directed life. Competency in self-care and homemaking skills may be attained by carrying out such activities oneself or by directing someone else who is employed to do so. Finally, the ability to establish and maintain close relationships may be demonstrated by being able to interact successfully with family, friends and personal care attendants (PCA).

Because self-care and homemaking skills have been considered a precursor of financial and emotional self-sufficiency and the establishment of a mature, intimate relationship, traditional medical rehabilitation, which focuses on eliminating or reducing physical impairments that interfere with self-care and homemaking activities, is seen as automatically providing IL services. Often, however, traditional medical rehabilitation fails to restore disabled people to their optimum level of independence, not because they are incapable but because traditional medical rehabilitation does not have the resources to do so (see Chapters 5 and 6).

**Basing Goals on Functional Deficits**  In traditional medical rehabilitation treatment objectives tend to be set by first categorizing people according to their disability type and then establishing goals for each type. People with cerebral palsy are viewed as requiring treatment primarily for their communication deficits and only secondarily for their mobility deficits (Hylbert and Hylbert, 1979). Those who are mentally retarded typically are given training in toileting and other basic self-care skills before being considered good candidates for academic training.

While few would argue that in setting training objectives for a severely retarded person toilet training is not important, problems arise when assessments of potential function are based on an existing mastery of self-care skills, rather than on categories of general deficits in basic living competencies.

In *Dummy* Tidyman (1974) relates the true story of Donald, an illiterate deaf-mute who was unable to defend himself against charges of murdering two young women. Because Donald was not toilet trained at an early age, he was denied admittance into a special education program in which he might have acquired some communication skills. Unable to read, write, or use sign language, he, nevertheless, under his mother's tutelage, learned to take care of himself and to handle his financial affairs, and was remuneratively employed on a loading dock.

An adult who acquires a spinal cord injury will also require toilet training, which will be relabeled as bowel and bladder management. In some instances training efforts are unsuccessful, and the adult will require help with his toileting routine for the rest of his life. In setting treatment objectives, however, in the case of an adventitiously disabled adult, failure in toilet training will not preclude the establishment of more advanced treatment goals, such as training for eventual employment.

Moreover, for physically disabled people in general there is no proven relationship between the accuracy of physicians' assessments of patients' physical function and the accuracy of their prognoses of eventual vocational and IL success (Margolin, 1971; Rubin and Roessler, 1978). Technological advances in functional aids or job engineering and modifications make it difficult for any professional to predict the self-care or job potential of any physically or mentally disabled individual unless the professional has done a specific ADL or work evaluation (Gold, 1975; Goldenson et al., 1978).

Severely disabled persons, that is, those functioning as quadriplegics because of rheumatoid arthritis, cerebral palsy, multiple sclerosis, muscular dystrophy, spinal cord injury, or poliomyelitis, have been successful in competitive employment in jobs ranging from the professional to the unskilled (Laurie, 1975, 1977; Mallik and Mueller, 1975). In terms of financial success, while there is a high percentage of unemployment and underemployment among disabled persons, a 1980 survey of disabled subscribers to "Accent on Living" revealed that 15 percent of those who responded had incomes of $30,000 or more; 20 percent had incomes from $20,000 to $29,000; 15 percent had incomes from $15,000 to $19,000; and 18 percent had incomes of $10,000 to $14,000. Although the readership of "Accent on Living" cannot be considered to be representative of disabled people in general, the results of the survey point out the fallacy of underestimating the potential of people with a variety of severely disabling conditions.

**Using Professional Resources**   In addition to guarding against inaccurate prognoses, it is important to arrive at treatment objectives that are based on the type, rather than the cause, of functional limitations. To a degree, a person with severe spastic cerebral palsy might be equated with a person with a high level of spinal cord injury during the goal-setting stage of IL services. At the outset both might be assumed to share a communication impairment as well as a mobility impairment. The person with cerebral palsy would lack the coordination to write without an assistive aid of some kind, while the person with a spinal cord injury would lack the hand and finger movement needed to write without an adaptive aid. Both might be better served if they were referred at the beginning to an expert in communication devices, rather than one being referred to a specialist in cerebral palsy and the other to a specialist in spinal cord injuries—specialists who might have only superficial knowledge of communication devices and techniques.

**Avoiding Functional Stereotypes** By initially using a functional framework, first to assess an individual's needs and then to match them with specifically prescribed services, professionals might avoid the tendency to prejudge clients in terms of the stereotypes associated with certain disability or age categories. It may be difficult for those who work only with elderly blind clients or young physically disabled clients to determine the degree to which client behaviors reflect the demand characteristics of an agency setting and the degree to which they reflect characteristics common to a particular age or disability group. To those who work with multiply handicapped children or adults, the diagnostic label "cerebral palsy" may be interpreted as referring to profoundly impaired people who require special seating before they can maintain an upright position. For them, "cerebral palsy" does not describe the condition of people who do not appear to have a disability until they attempt a task requiring fine eye-hand coordination.

A neurologist who specializes in multiple sclerosis (MS) believes the distress newly diagnosed patients experience is intensified because they share the mistaken but widely held belief that MS is invariably a rapidly progressing, totally incapacitating disorder. In fact, according to this neurologist, the majority of his patients display no visible manifestation of their neurological disorder and suffer no disruption in their daily lives.

Independent living rehabilitation (ILR), because it is designed to improve individuals' ability to direct their own lives and decrease their dependence on others, depends on precise analyses of clients' function, independent of age or disability type. In ILR, client labels such as "high risk" are inappropriate. In traditional vocational rehabilitation, a "high-risk" client is one whose eventual employability is in doubt because of age, severity of disability, poor general health, or lack of stamina. Unlike traditional vocational rehabilitation, where rehabilitative success is clearly defined as eventual job placement, ILR has no potentially "high-risk" clients. The concept of optimum independence means that IL services might be effective if they result in a bedridden person being able to use a telephone effectively enough for family members to be freed from the need for 24-hour-a-day supervision.

The 1978 Amendments, by authorizing services that "improve significantly" an individual's "ability to function independently in his family or community," provided the opportunity to eliminate some of the resource- and money-wasting barriers that segregate people receiving educational and rehabilitation services according to their age or disability type. As long as providers of services to disabled children must vie for funds and public support with providers of services to disabled adults, as long as providers of services to the mentally retarded must vie with providers of services to the blind, needless man-hours and energy will be expended in the struggle for territory and professional survival. If fully implemented, the 1978 Amendments, by not excluding any rehabilitative goals, would ensure that funds and services were better spent to meet the rehabilitation needs of all disabled people, regardless of age or disability type. Reallocating funds from existing service delivery systems that provide overlapping services to disabled people would support training for IL specialists, for the operation of IL programs, and for carrying out outreach and follow-up procedures that would ensure that those presently living below their optimum levels of functioning would receive the services they require to live more independently.

## MAINTAINING OPTIMUM INDEPENDENCE

Once people have attained the IL goals compatible with their mental and physical capabilities and limitations, intermittent IL services will usually be necessary if they are to maintain this optimum level. There are many factors that, if not controlled, contribute to the decline of hard-won IL skills.

**Lack of Follow-up Services**  The period immediately following the conclusion of intensive IL services is critical. Without periodic reinforcement, mentally retarded people have been found to lose their ability to prepare and select appropriate foods (Knight, 1980). Physically disabled people may revert to passive or physically dependent behaviors when families or friends continue to regard and treat them as though they were still incapable of functioning more independently. Deterioration of independent behaviors may, in turn, precipitate health problems that might have been avoided if client behaviors had been monitored periodically and retraining had been instituted when necessary.

**Secondary Disabilities**  Physically disabled persons are prone to develop habits that may enhance functioning in the short run but impede their ability to function over a longer period. When Peter S., an SCI quadriplegic, found he could transfer to and from his wheelchair more easily if he bent his back, he also discovered that hunching his shoulders helped him maintain his balance while he was sitting in his wheelchair. Eventually, Peter developed a severe abnormal curvature of the upper spine that interfered with his respiration and his ability to drive his car long distances.

Disabled people, as they get older, are subject to secondary disabilities—disabilities that arise as a normal consequence of aging or a prior disability. Many secondary disabilities are avoidable and originate from disuse or misuse of the body. All secondary disabilities complicate the attempts of disabled people to live more independently.

Like the general population, mentally retarded people, even if their sight and hearing are not already affected, will eventually develop presbyopia (diminished clarity of vision due to aging) and presbycusis (diminished acuity of hearing due to aging). People who acquire a physical disability early in life may also, through the normal aging process, acquire a degenerative disability—high blood pressure, emphysema, osteoarthritis, and so on. Osteoarthritis, the arthritic condition that stems from the normal degeneration of weight-bearing joints over time, may occur at a much earlier age in those with disabilities that force them to overuse certain areas of their bodies, such as the arms and shoulders in the case of paraplegics.

Beth P., who works at CIL, used a manual wheelchair and drove a car equipped with handcontrols when she was a student at the University of Illinois. She is currently using an electric wheelchair and is driving a modified van, which she operates from her wheelchair. Beth has adopted mobility aids that are used by more severely disabled people because she began to experience repeated episodes of pain, numbness, and loss of function in her arms and hands from muscle spasms that compressed her cervical nerves. After she began using mobility aids that did not require the continual use of her neck and shoulder muscles, the episodes of pain, numbness, and loss of function did not recur.

While some degenerative processes can be prevented or delayed by a change in the techniques or devices a person uses, others are unavoidable. In either case rehabilitative and educational measures should be instituted to enable disabled people of any age to cope with any physical changes and to help them maintain what physical function they can. In addition to training clients in behaviors that will prevent certain secondary disabilities from occurring, IL specialists who periodically monitor the progress of former clients will be in a position to detect incipient functional problems and either alert the clients or their physicians or institute another round of IL services.

**Disuse Secondary Disabilities**   Disuse secondary disabilities are disabilities that occur because of inactivity. They most often affect skeletal tissue and joints. Two common disuse secondary disabilities are obesity and atrophy.

*Obesity*   A person becomes obese when he or she eats more food than the body requires and excess food products are stored as fatty tissue. Disabled people become obese when their activity levels drop dramatically, as when an athlete is paralyzed and begins to use an electric wheelchair without changing his or her eating habits. Obesity among the disabled may also stem from overeating because of boredom, anxiety, or poor eating habits. Wolfensberger (1980) cites the craving many mentally retarded people have for foods high in carbohydrates. Some disabled people with limited food budgets may buy foods that are high in calories but relatively inexpensive, such as peanut butter or beans. Difficulty with food preparation may also contribute to an increase in weight because prepackaged, canned, or frozen meals contain a high proportion of flour and sugar compared to similar foods prepared at home.

Adam P., who is 26 and has spastic cerebral palsy, was 40 pounds overweight. The first year he lived alone he subsisted on pastries, hamburgers, and french fries he bought at a small coffee shop close to his apartment. According to Adam, convenience food is something one can buy and heat in a container that can then be thrown away. After Adam began working as a computer programmer, he bought an electric frying pan, which he used on his dining room table. Later he added a microwave oven to his cooking area and perfected a variety of low-calorie, one-dish meals that he could prepare easily and safely. He avoided the need to use sharp knives by purchasing chopped or sliced frozen fruits and vegetables. Eventually, Adam experienced an improvement in both his weight and his social life, since he often invited friends over for dinner. What Adam learned by himself through a long process of trial and error he could have learned in one or two sessions of a homemaking module offered by many IL programs as part of their service package.

In any IL program, it is important to address the subject of appropriate eating habits. According to Hirshberg, Lewis, and Vaughn (1976), what would normally be a reducing diet might cause a weight gain in a physically disabled person. Hirshberg et al. state that disabled people may have to restrict their daily calorie intake to 600 or 400 calories in order to achieve a weight loss or to maintain their weight at a desirable level. These low daily calorie intakes, with mineral and vitamin supplements, will meet a person's nutritional needs, these researchers claim, and can be achieved if the person is prepared to accept a breakfast restricted to the white of an egg and a cup of unsweetened tea (Hirshberg et al., 1976).

For many disabled people who are precluded from the usual stress-reducing activities—drinking, smoking, and heavy physical exercise—food assumes an unusually important role, psychologically as well as physiologically. Recognition of the need for training in weight control and good nutritional habits has always played a role in the services offered by outstanding medical rehabilitation facilities. When polio was still prevalent, the staff on what was then the Georgia Warm Springs Foundation conducted weekly weigh-ins of all patients, placed them on diets tailored to meet their needs, and schooled them in the importance of maintaining a prescribed body weight to maximize the functional capacity of their weakened muscles. Independent living programs, through training in food preparation and nutrition and through sponsorship of client support groups, can directly address the area of weight control.

*Atrophy*   Atrophy occurs when muscle mass diminishes because of insufficient innervation of muscle fibers. Its precipitating cause is inactivity or disuse of muscle fibers. While atrophy is unavoidable in conditions like muscular dystrophy, where normal muscle tissue is replaced by fatty and connective tissue through the disease process, or like polio, where the nerve supply to the muscle is destroyed, avoidable atrophy can be as disabling as the primary disabling condition. Before people who have had strokes can walk, when one leg remains functionally limited by spastic paralysis, they must develop and maintain the strength of muscles in the unaffected side of their bodies. When the unaffected side is strong, they will be able to rise to a standing position from a sitting position and will be able to ambulate with a walker, a cane, or no mobility aid at all. Similarly, it is important for paraplegics, quadriplegics, and amputees to develop strength in their unimpaired muscles, if they are to function as independently as they otherwise might.

**Misuse Secondary Disabilities**  The second major category of secondary disabilities that can result in a renewed need for IL services is disabilities that result from inappropriate use of the body. Misuse disabilities stem from improper self-care or the acquisition of habits that initially simplify daily living routines but that, over time, create additional physical limitations.

*Decubitus Ulcers (Pressure Sores)*  A common and potentially life-threatening misuse secondary disability is the decubitus ulcer, or pressure sore. Decubitus ulcers occur when a person who has a loss of sensation or who has difficulty shifting body positions remains in one position too long. This cuts off or reduces the blood supply to a weight-bearing portion of the body, resulting in the death of body tissues. The areas of the skin lying over the tail bone, shoulder blades, hip bones, the ischial tuberosities, elbows, heels, and knees are common sites for pressure sores, because there is little fat or muscle tissue cushioning the bony prominances in these areas.

In order to prevent pressure sores, people with severe sensory or mobility impairments must learn to shift their weight periodically and to check daily for signs of tissue destruction. Those who are incapable of shifting their own positions must rely on the assistance of others to ensure that ulceration does not occur. According to Hirshberg et al. (1976), people who are confined to bed and who can't position or pad themselves should be turned every half-hour because tissue destruction can result from unrelieved pressure in 30 minutes. Prevention is important because once the skin ulcerates, the ulcers heal slowly and, in some instances, become chronic or incurable. Since treatment for pressure sores, in addition to keeping the area clean and exposed to light and air, is the total elimination of pressure from the affected area, decubitus ulcers can reduce people who were self-sufficient to bedfast dependency.

*Other Misuse Disabilities*  Although decubitus ulcers are one of the most potentially incapacitating, there are many other misuse disabilities. Loss of vision and loss of the lower extremities are not uncommon misuse disabilities in people with diabetes, although for many they are unavoidable consequences of long-term diabetes.

Similarly, while many persons with rheumatoid arthritis become incapacitated because of an uncontrollable progression of the disease, others lose function unnecessarily because they do not use splinting devices that would correct or forestall their deformities. For example, leg braces may counteract the effect of progressive destruction of structures supporting the knee joint, which if untreated will produce a condition known as "backward knee," in which the knee joint becomes permanently hyperextended.

Misuse disabilities can erode the success of the best rehabilitation program, unless some method is available to detect and prevent their occurrence. Independent living services, by providing additional training in self-care and periodic client follow-up, can help avert these disabilities before they develop to the point where they impede individuals' attempts to care for themselves.

## SOCIAL INTEGRATION

A fundamental goal of the IL paradigm is that the disabled be integrated into society as completely as possible. This goal, however, is not achieved by ensuring that the elderly disabled can continue to live in their own homes or by transferring younger disabled people out of institutions into community-based housing. To be truly integrated, disabled persons must be able not only to live within their own communities, but also to enjoy the privileges and assume the responsibilities of community living.

Federal legislation and court decisions based on existing legislation (see Chapter 1), extending back to *Brown* v. *The Board of Education* and the 1978 Amendments to the 1973 Rehabilitation Act, establish both the right of disabled people to participate in the activities and the benefits of the wider society and the means through which they can do so (DeLoach and Greer, 1981). The role of social integration in establishing IL goals differs in the United States from some other countries that also provide rehabilitation services, but at the cost of the autonomy and privacy of those who are physically disabled (Wolfensberger, 1978). Oftentimes, however, differences in the preferred mode of service delivery are more practical than philosophical. Terrain in mountainous countries, architecture in older sections of European and Asian cities, and longstanding customs in many places often prevent environmental accessibility and foster a passive dependency that militates against successful integration of the world's more than 450 million visibly disabled people (Laurie, 1977). In her book *Housing and Home Services for the Disabled*, Laurie outlines the advantages of living in a country as diverse as the United States with its varying climates and terrain and its wide range in styles of architecture. Here disabled persons, providing they are free to move, can select areas of the country that best suit their type of disability. Choices are more limited in countries like Malaysia, where rural homes are built on stilts, making them impossible to ramp conveniently, and where free-standing latrines have door sills as high as windows, ensuring that snakes as well as humans with severe mobility impairments cannot enter. Even if these structures had accessible entrances, mobility impaired people still could not function without assistance, for in areas such as these the "plumbing" consists of an opening in the subflooring that allows water to drain into a "soak pit" underneath the structure.

In Australia, too, for example, the concept of independent living is more restricted than here. The function of Australian IL centers is limited to the collection, evaluation, and dissemination of assistive devices (Parameter, 1980). In the United States, the absence of a national health program, which provides disabled citizens with transportation, housing, medical and attendant services, means that the variety of support services that are necessary for the optimum independent functioning of disabled persons becomes the responsibility, in theory at least, of the IL programs. The programs either provide these services directly or work to coordinate services that are provided by other social programs and agencies. According to the Seventh Institute on Rehabilitation Issues (1980), "any Independent Living Program that is established should offer the following core services: information and referral, financial benefits, counseling, peer counseling, transportation and attendant referral." The ways in which the different types of IL programs provide these core services, in addition to other services, such as housing, will be discussed in Parts Two and Three.


## LEVELS OF INDEPENDENCE

In countries such as Australia, IL services are designed primarily to attain the first two of three levels of independent functioning that are necessary to the optimum social integration of disabled people. These levels are (1) independence in bed, (2) independence in the home, and (3) independence in the community.


### INDEPENDENCE IN BED

Someone who has attained independence in bed, according to Hirshberg et al. (1976), is capable of feeding, bathing, and dressing him- or herself in addition to being able to use a bedpan or urinal without assistance. People who are limited to this level of physical independence are usually those with disabilities where cardiovascular or respiratory restrictions severely limit their activity levels or where dependence on a life support system restricts their mobility. At this level of independence, a disabled person has to have someone else prepare, serve, and clear away meals, bring bathwater and toilet articles, and empty and clean bathroom utensils. This degree of assistance requires little strength or skill, however, so that a child, an elderly parent or spouse, or another disabled person can easily provide what assistance is necessary. At this level of physical independence, family members are freed from rigorous nursing duties and can engage in activities outside the home, because the person who is disabled can be left alone for reasonable periods, as long as some provision is made so that help can be summoned in an emergency.

## INDEPENDENCE IN THE HOME

At this level of independence, the disabled may move about freely inside the home by using a power or manual wheelchair, a walker, or no mobility aid at all. Independence at this level entails the ability to dress, bathe, and groom oneself, and to transfer to and from the bed and the commode. The disabled person may or may not be self-sufficient in food preparation or housekeeping tasks, and, if he or she is not, will require housekeeper and shopping services. In many sections of the country, a minimum of one hot meal a day is delivered to a disabled person's home under the auspices of a variety of privately or publicly sponsored programs, such as Meals on Wheels. Social contacts and help in emergencies can be provided through telephone services.

Today, many people are confined to this intermediate level of independent functioning because they live in inaccessible housing or lack accessible means of transportation. Such people lead lives that are more limited than they would be if the people lived in barrier-free homes and communities.

## INDEPENDENCE IN THE COMMUNITY

At this third level of independence, people are able to move about within their communities without assistance. Such people live in accessible housing. In addition, they drive privately owned modified vehicles or have access to barrier-free public transportation, which allows them to engage in social activities outside their homes, to participate in community affairs and, if they are employed, to get to and from their jobs.

## OVERLAPPING LEVELS

A paradox becomes evident when IL behaviors are classified according to the levels of independence described above. As medical treatment and the technology that produces adaptive aids and assistive devices advance, it becomes increasingly common for persons who are not independent at levels one and two to be totally independent at level three. Someone who may be dependent while in bed may, once placed in a wheelchair, require no further assistance until he or she is returned to bed. People of this kind, if the environment in which they live is appropriately arranged, may, with the aid of assistive devices, prepare meals, do light housecleaning and laundry, and drive a modified van (Gilbert, 1973). Many such people are active within their communities, often serving as volunteers, even though they continue to require assistance from others for brief intervals during the day (Deyoe, 1972).

Before IL programs can provide services that increase the ability of severely disabled persons to live more independently, service providers must first identify the levels at which new clients are currently functioning. Then they must determine what services are needed to increase clients' levels of functioning. And, finally, they must coordinate needed services that are already available, or, if possible, provide those that are not available.

Because full social participation by disabled people depends on their having access to barrier-free housing, transportation, medical care facilities, and recreational and job sites, IL services cannot be considered apart from a wide network of community-wide support services. In Parts Two and Three the community services upon which IL programs must depend will be discussed in detail.

## THE CONCEPT OF NORMALIZATION

The final overall goal of IL services is to assist severely disabled people of all ages to attain lifestyles that do not differ substantially from those of their nondisabled contemporaries. The process of assisting disabled people to lead lives that are as "normal" as possible is termed normalization, and normalization is the underlying principle of the IL movement.

The concept of normalization originated as a paradigm of treatment and services that were designed to assist mentally retarded people to lead lives that were as normal and self-fulfilling as possible. As two leading theorists of the normalization movement, Wolfensberger (1972, 1980) and Nirje (1969, 1980), point out, the intent of normalization is not to eliminate physical and mental differences among individuals. Instead, its overriding goal is to moderate the differences in lifestyle and living opportunities that disabled people experience because of their inability to merge into social living patterns without some special accommodations being made for them. Normalization does not have as its goal, however, that elderly disabled people should become young again or live the style of life of nondisabled elderly people. Rather, normalization means that the elderly disabled should be able to lead lives equal in quality to the lives of others—that is, they should be able to continue to live in their own homes, enjoy the company of their friends, be secure financially, be able to engage in a variety of satisfying avocational or vocational pursuits, and, generally, lead the life they choose to lead.

The principle of normalization helps to clarify what types of IL services are most appropriate for what groups of persons. When the principle of normalization is used as a gauge, successful outcomes for IL services can be described as those where not only are people integrated into society, but their patterns of living are similar to those of their nondisabled contemporaries.

Housing is an example often used to illustrate the concept of normalized lifestyles or patterns. Because "normal" children live in families consisting of one or more children and one or two consistent parental figures, according to the principle of normalization, disabled children should live in their parental or foster homes. They should not be placed in settings where the ratio of children to adults and the on-site living conditions differ drastically from what is normal for nondisabled children. Because in our society young adults typically move out of their parents' homes to establish homes of their own, service policies that reflect the normalization principle would attempt to place young disabled adults into one-person living units or pair them with one or two compatible room- or apartment-mates. Finally, because elderly people tend to live apart from their children and other family members, away from the constant company of small children, normalization policies would result in elderly disabled people remaining in their homes or being placed in living situations that best replicate what they would have chosen had they had no need of IL services.

The goals that independent living, as a social service paradigm, is designed to achieve are, unfortunately, beyond the scope of existing services. Nevertheless, even present IL services could affect every aspect of the lives of disabled people by restructuring them into as "normal" a mode as possible. IL services, however, as authorized by the 1978 Amendments and as offered through the grass-roots IL programs, cannot be used to best advantage while severely disabled people do not have access to barrier-free private or public transportation (see Chapter 8). For example, few people today, even with a resurgence of cottage industries, receive their education or are employed at the site where they live. Institutions or congregate living centers in which educational facilities and job sites are contained within the same complex, therefore, are not "normal." Such facilities and sites may not, however, be avoidable if those with mobility impairments continue to lack reliable, affordable, and accessible transport.

## GENERIC VERSUS SPECIFIC SERVICES

It is important to remember that independence is a relative concept, whether a person is disabled or not. Independent living services are not designed to transform functionally limited people into totally physically self-sufficient superbeings. While increased physical self-sufficiency is always a goal, success can be attained by moving people who require services through a series of intermediate goals to a level of physical, and interpersonal, functioning that is judged optimal by both professionals who provide the IL services and the individuals who receive them. Just as independence has many variations in the IL paradigm, degrees of functional independence, too, are variable, liable to shift with each marked change in life's circumstances, before once again stabilizing in a temporary balance of dependent and independent behaviors. Success in attaining IL objectives can best be assessed by first determining whether an individual's level of functional ability increased and, second, by determining how long he or she maintained that increased level. Given the nature of physical disabilities, any dramatic alteration in a disabled person's health or living situation can create the need for an additional functional assessment and, perhaps, an additional round of prescribed services.

Independent living has never had as a goal the ability to train and equip persons so they could live without assistance, but isolated from the stream of daily activities in their communities.

The goal of social integration is not to bring disabled people to the point where they can participate in every activity and behave in exactly the same way as do those who are not disabled; the goal is to mold the daily living patterns of those with disabilities as much as possible into the daily living patterns of their nondisabled contemporaries.

The following cases illustrate the basic principles of independent living, which are that (1) there is a need for some generic services that are not restricted to people of a particular age or disability type, (2) services should be determined and provided according to the unique needs of each disabled individual, and (3) the determinants of success in independent living should be based both on increasing an individual's ability to function independently and on maintaining an individual's ability to function at his or her optimum level of independence for as long as possible.

---

## CASE ONE: ELEANOR M.

Eleanor, an 84-year-old widow who lived alone in a neighborhood of elderly people, began to experience severe pain in her left hip and thigh. After a year of self-medication, with increasing discomfort, she consulted an orthopedic surgeon who diagnosed *malum coxae senilis* (diseased hip of the aging) and recommended a total hip replacement.

Following her corrective surgery, Eleanor spent three weeks in a general medical hospital but was still unable to get in and out of bed, dress, bathe, or walk down the hall without assistance. Because she lived alone and had no one to help her with her personal care, her housework, or her grocery shopping, Eleanor was transferred to a nursing home instead of being allowed to return to her home as she had requested.

Once in the nursing home, which was understaffed, Eleanor discovered that there was seldom anyone available to help her in and out of bed or walk up and down the hall with her. After an additional three weeks of convalescence, during which she made no appreciable gains in strength or self-care skills, Eleanor developed phlebitis and was transferred back to the general medical hospital. By the time the phlebitis cleared up, Eleanor had made arrangements of her own that made it possible for her to return home instead of to the nursing facility. Two of her neighbors had agreed to share her housecleaning and shopping chores, a senior citizens group agreed to deliver her meals, and a public health nurse was to visit her daily to help her with her personal care.

Once she was home, Eleanor gained strength quickly, due to a series of exercises she learned from the nurse. By the time she had been home for a month, she was adept in the use of her walker and could do all her own cooking and light housecleaning. Today, four years after her surgery, Eleanor continues to live alone. Although she walks with a slight limp, she still tends her vegetable garden and continues to play an active role in her church and senior citizens group. She is, however, experiencing increasing discomfort in her right hip and thigh and in both knees.

## CASE TWO: SUSAN J.

A multiply handicapped 8-year-old, Susan attends a special school for severely disabled children, but has not learned to read or write and is totally dependent on others for her personal care. Susan's mother and father, while concerned about the day-to-day problems of caring for Susan—they haven't found a way to eliminate her strong underarm odor and are already wondering about the best way to handle her menstrual flow—worry most about what will happen to Susan as they grow older, or if they die before she does. Although both parents have developed back problems, they often must lift and carry their daughter, who continues to increase in size and body weight. Although they would prefer to keep Susan at home, they are investigating the possibility of placing her in an institution. They are afraid that if they don't find a place for her soon, they may be unable to find an institution that will accept her when they may no longer be able to care for her. A developmental center near their home has 500 residents, has a long waiting list, and is currently trying to decrease the overall number of residents by not accepting any new admissions and by moving the more capable residents into group or foster homes. Susan's mother says she often wakes up in the middle of the night trembling and crying, fearful of what might happen to her daughter someday.

Susan's parents have received some valuable assistance from a rehabilitation engineering center about 100 miles from their home. Several devices the center developed specially for them have made it easier for them to handle Susan. For example, although tub baths reduce Susan's spasticity, her parents were beginning to find it difficult to lift her in and out of the tub and to keep her head above the water when strong extensor spasms in her back forced her head toward the bottom of the tub. The center's staff devised a tub insert that supports Susan's head and shoulders, but that still allows the rest of her body to be immersed. The staff also designed a modular wheelchair that greatly simplifies the process of transferring Susan into and out of the car and on and off the commode.

## CASE THREE: ERNIE C.

A 19-year-old who became a quadriplegic in a fall from a trapeze bar in a high-school gym, Ernie recently became engaged. After his injury, Ernie received acute medical care in a general medical hospital and then was transferred to a rehabilitation hospital, where he learned to dress, bathe, manage his own bowel and bladder care, and drive a car equipped with hand controls. What Ernie lacked most after his medical rehabilitation was a usable vocational skill, but during the time he was actively engaged in the medical rehabilitation process, he refused any further schooling, career counseling, or vocational training. Neither was he interested in learning any homemaking or home management skills. Since he was going to live with his parents, he reasoned, his mother could continue to do the cooking, cleaning, and laundry as before.

Then Ernie met Ruth, who is in nurses' training. Ruth wants to marry Ernie but has made it very clear she expects to be his wife, not his nurse. Moreover, she expects Ernie to do his share of the routine housekeeping chores. Now that living with his parents has lost its appeal, Ernie desperately wants to find a job and an accessible apartment, and to learn some homemaking skills. Above all, Ernie is obsessed with the desire to establish a home of his own, free from what has become an onerous dependence on his parents.

## CASE FOUR: MARIE S.

For the past 43 years, Marie, who has been diagnosed as mentally retarded, has been living in an institution that has recently been retitled as a developmental center. The center's new director has taken an interest in Marie's case and views her as a challenge to his ability to move long-term residents into the community. Convinced that her disability is as much emotional as intellectual, he believes Marie has learned to mimic the physical posturings and interpersonal behaviors of the more severely retarded residents.

Only recently has Marie been diagnosed as having a hearing impairment that, while it could be due to the normal aging process, could have been responsible for her lack of language skills.

At present, however, Marie resists not only the idea that she might leave the center but also any attempt to take her outside of the center's grounds. When she was placed in a community skills training group, she became withdrawn, almost catatonic. The one time she nearly left the center was when a volunteer, who had become a special friend of Marie's, received permission to take Marie home for a weekend. Marie agreed to go, entered her friend's car willingly, but as soon as the car drove through the gates, became agitated and nearly succeeded in jumping out of the moving vehicle. Fearing Marie would hurt herself, the friend turned around and brought Marie back.

The cases above illustrate (1) the range of services that may be required to enhance the IL potential of persons with various functional deficits and (2) the range in ages of those who could benefit from IL services. In each case, as research has demonstrated, an individual's motivation is basic to the success or failure of rehabilitation (Thorenson et al., 1968; Chapter 13). Eleanor's desire to remain in her own home has played a major role in her being able to continue living alone for as long as she has. Ernie's desire to marry provided an incentive for him to leave the responsibility-free life he leads with his parents. Marie, however, is strongly motivated to remain dependent and is unwilling to exchange whatever security she feels for what might await her in the community. In Susan's case, it is her parents' motivation to provide for their daughter's future that fuels the drive to seek out the services and devices that will lessen the difficulties of caring for Susan. In Chapter 9 further parallels, as well as differences, will be drawn among these four cases to illustrate how IL services can enhance the lives of a variety of people, whatever the degree of their physical limitations or in whatever living situation they find themselves.

# 3

## Matching Community Resources and Personal Capabilities

In these last decades of the twentieth century, independent living, as a social service innovation, is in a critical phase of its evolution (Flynn and Nitsch, 1980). Long-awaited, and supported by a majority of disabled people and rehabilitation professionals, the concept of independent living and an independent living service delivery system was finally granted legislative recognition on the federal level through Title VII, Parts A, B, C, and D of the 1978 Amendments to the 1973 Rehabilitation Act (see Chapter 1). But as with any social service philosophy that has just passed the hurdle of legislative legitimation, independent living then reached the crucible of implementation. This critical phase occurred during the massive cutbacks in government-sponsored social service programs of the early 1980s. Whether or not the systematized services, which allow severely disabled persons to live as full a life as possible, continue to exist on a nationwide basis depends on empirical proof that IL programs are effective. Before the IL service delivery system can become widely implemented, programs will have to prove their economic utility, as well as their humanitarian value. Otherwise, the requisite diversion of funds from existing social service channels will not take place. In view of the overall reduction of monies for human services, reallocation is likely to be the only way that IL services will acquire adequate funding.

As with any social innovation, it is easier to explain the concept of independent living than it is to determine the most feasible method for translating the concept into an effective social service delivery system. Institutionalization is rendered even more difficult by the diversity of acceptable IL goals (see Chapter 2). But if independent living, as a social service system, is institutionalized, IL services may potentially affect the lives of 29 million disabled people of all ages, especially the 15 million who have severe and permanently incapacitating conditions (National Center for Health Statistics, 1977).

Even though progress is slow, however, viable modes of delivering services are being developed. In 1980, 60 government grants of $200,000 each were awarded to state divisions of vocational rehabilitation or, when state divisions did not apply, to private agencies. These grants were designed to establish IL projects that would serve as models for future projects within each state. Even before these 60 projects were established through federal funding, however, over 200 IL centers and programs were already in operation, several for nearly 10 years. Although subject to strict government guidelines, the 60 projects begun in 1980, like those established earlier, featured a variety of service formats.

The range of services offered by IL programs is striking in view of the fact that most programs are designed to assist two general categories of disabled people—the mentally retarded and young people with mobility impairments (ILRUP, 1979). Independent living programs that existed prior to the 1980s evidenced little interest in providing services to people with visual or hearing impairments or the elderly disabled. Whether this focus on the mentally retarded and the mobility impaired was because these groups have a greater need for services, because they have a more visible need for services, or because many of the earlier programs for the young physically disabled were founded by paraplegics and quadriplegics is difficult to determine.

At a time when the competition among the various groups of human service providers for decreasing funds is increasing, it is imperative that IL services be rendered according to areas of greatest need rather than areas where needs are most easily met. Those who are dedicated to meeting the needs of disabled people remember that before the 1973 mandate to serve the severely disabled, many who eventually learned to live independently and found employment were unable to obtain assistance from state vocational rehabilitation agencies. Before the 1973 Rehabilitation Act, vocational rehabilitation services were more readily available to so-called low-risk people—who would in any case have found employment more easily—than to high-risk people with severely incapacitating conditions, who found it difficult to be determined eligible for the training and placement services that would have helped them reenter the community.

This chapter will

1. explore the two contradictory philosophies of independent living,

2. delineate the categories of services offered by each type of IL program;

3. identify the factors that determine the type of services that a particular program offers,

4. discuss the different competency areas that professionals have identified as being essential to optimum independence for clients.

## TWO OPPOSING VIEWS
## OF INDEPENDENT LIVING

Chapter 2 discussed what the goal of independent living is not, namely, the transformation of disabled persons into totally independent superbeings. As exaggerated as this view of independent living might seem, it is not too different from one of the prevailing philosophies of independent living. To clarify this philosophy and the goals it suggests, the authors call this orientation the society-oriented philosophy of independent living.

### THE SOCIETY-ORIENTED PHILOSOPHY
### OF INDEPENDENT LIVING

The society-oriented philosophy of independent living, as evidenced in the Illinois model, appears to have originated as an overreaction to the misconception that people who have a physical incapacity are, as a consequence, incapacitated in every other area as well. As elucidated in Parsons' (1958) theory of social roles, this misconception holds that (1) disability is synonymous with illness, or, in other words, people who are disabled are sick, and (2) their sickness prevents them from carrying out any of their expected social roles.

According to Parsons' theory, illness creates a situation in which society demands a ritualistic response from those who have become ill. While illness, within limits, exempts people from the demands of their usual roles, the state of being ill is only conditionally sanctioned within a culture that recognizes health as the only natural—that is, "good"—state. Within our culture, states Parsons, sympathy and exoneration from work and familial responsibilities are granted only if a person recognizes and admits that his illness is an undesirable state and cooperates with others to actively seek out and submit to whatever treatment is prescribed to restore him to a healthy, "desirable" state. Illness is considered to be an invariably temporary condition *if* the person who is ill upholds the correct cultural values and carries out the appropriate remedial measures. An individual, therefore, will receive special consideration—that is, sympathy and exoneration from responsibilities—for only a limited time, during which he must admit that his condition is totally undesirable and actively strive to regain his capacity for "independent achievement and economic productivity."

What happens, then, when an illness is chronic, or when an accident, illness, or congenital condition results in a permanent physical impairment? Because society has no clear-cut social mechanism for incorporating that person or that person's situation into existing, acceptable social roles, the physically disabled person, along with the delinquent and the addict, is labeled and treated as a deviant member of society. This means that for as long as the disability persists the person will be subject to pressure—medical, social, psychological, and religious—to recover his lost physical capacity. In short, he will be expected, according to the society-oriented philosophy of independent living, to compensate for his deviant state by striving to perform his usual social roles, irrespective of whether or not this is possible or feasible.

According to McDaniel (1976), society is not only concerned with maintaining and controlling the social capacities of its members, but also works to forestall or rectify any disturbances in their capacities. The meaning of this for disabled people varies to some degree from one society to another and from one historical period to another. Although at any one time in any society a wide range of attitudes and behaviors toward disabled people exists, certain types of attitudes and behaviors tend to predominate. At present, in our society, researchers have discovered that voiced attitudes toward the disabled are mildly positive, while unvoiced attitudes range from mildly negative to deeply hostile (Roessler and Bolton, 1978).

Within the Western world, five general trends in societal attitudes toward and treatment of the chronically ill and disabled, each predominant in a historical period, have been identified by Kolstoe and Frey (1965). The first period, which they call the Era of Extermination, was in ancient times when the effect of superstitious explanations for the occurrence of disability, combined with concern for survival of the human species, was a largely routine destruction of disabled people, especially disabled newborns. Recent evidence indicates, however, that fewer defective infants were destroyed in ancient Sparta and Rome than was formerly supposed, and that some congenital disabilities were considered to be desirable traits by ancient peoples. For example, the birth of a child with a harelip was thought to be a sign of good fortune in an early Roman household (Fiedler, 1978).

In the second period, entitled the Era of Ridicule, people with disabilities attained a marginal acceptance, sometimes making their living by performing as court jesters or as attractions in freak shows.

The third period, the Era of Asylum, occurred during the Middle Ages, when some private (often religion-based) and public provisions were made for the sustenance and shelter of those with physical and mental impairments. Often, however, it appears from descriptions of places designed to house the disabled or the mentally ill, or from the paintings of Goya (1746–1828), that these asylums were less places of refuge than places of punishment and restriction.

The fourth period, the Era of Education, typified much of the eighteenth and nineteenth centuries, in which many schools and training programs for the blind, the deaf, and the mentally retarded were established. By the end of the nineteenth century, however, many of these educationally based institutions had turned into institutions whose primary function was the administration of lifelong custodial care, not only to provide for those who were deemed incapable of caring for themselves, but also to protect society from deviants who must otherwise return to their homes and communities.

The final major trend in attitudes toward and treatment of the disabled, according to Kolstoe and Frey (1965), is reflected in the Era of Occupational Adequacy or Vocational Rehabilitation (Payne, Mercer, and Epstein, 1974). In this era, which continues to the present, the predominant philosophy concerning the disabled is that they should be provided with a full range of educational, medical, and community services so that they can become participating members of society.

Proponents of the society-based philosophy of independent living believe that, given medical and technological advances that minimize or eradicate the handicapping effects of many disabling conditions, disabled people are obligated to assume their share of societal responsibilities, at whatever personal cost. These proponents believe that each disabled person has a duty to other disabled people to attempt to reduce the social stigma of disability by proving that being disabled does not preclude one from being a productive member of society. They fear that, unless the social status of disabled people improves, the progressive devaluation of human life in general may result in a renewed Era of Extermination for those whose lives are already seen as having little societal value (DeLoach and Greer, 1981; Dowd and Emner, 1978; Fiedler, 1978; Ramsey, 1978; Stein, 1978).

## THE INDIVIDUAL-ORIENTED PHILOSOPHY OF INDEPENDENT LIVING

The second major philosophical orientation toward independent living is best described as an individual-oriented philosophy. Proponents of this orientation believe that control by the individual over his or her own life is the ultimate goal of IL services, since self-determination is the basic component of a truly independent lifestyle. Therefore, proponents of this orientation consider functional independence—the physical ability to be self-sufficient in self-care and homemaking activities—to be, in many instances, detrimental to an optimally independent lifestyle, as, for example, when carrying out these activities without assistance requires so much time and energy that little is left for other activities (Laurie, 1977). This orientation emphasizes an individual's right to choose, even if he or she exercises that right by choosing to remain physically or economically dependent. Andrea C., a quadriplegic who writes, "To me, independence is the freedom to survey all of the available alternatives in a given situation and then use this collected information to make a conscious choice," concludes, ". . . for now, I prefer to depend upon a person pushing me rather than an electric chair" (Cappaert, 1979, p. 25).

Dart, Dart, and Nosek (1980) describe what they believe are the effects of evaluating success in independent living in terms of how physically independent a person becomes:

We must not make the mistake of sacrificing control and quality of life for an inflexible adherence to certain symbols, methods, definitions and situations that may for some present only a facade of living independently. The dogmatic thrusting of expensive, possibly unsatisfying and often unreachable goals on individuals can have a devastating effect. When the attainment of a positive self-image is dependent on the achievement of that which cannot be achieved or maintained, or cannot be maintained without the making of self-defeating sacrifices, then waste, frustration and unnecessary subjugation to authority, and perceptions of a lower overall quality of life result. Instead of becoming increasingly independent, the individual becomes self-destructively dependent, much the same as the individual in a developing country who is influenced to give up a relatively fulfilling and secure "primitive" culture in order to acquire certain material and psychosocial symbols of modernism which are frequently beyond his or her grasp, and are often impractical and/or unsatisfying when acquired. (P. 17)

Interestingly, the drive to become and remain more physically self-sufficient appears to correspond less with severity of disability than with how much assistance a person is accustomed to receiving (DeLoach and Greer, 1981; Hitz, 1980). Employees of VA hospitals remark that married spinal cord injured (SCI) veterans are often more dependent than unmarried SCI veterans with the same degree of impairment.

As outlined in the previous chapter, programs that provide IL services must consider the severity of the clients' disability, the degree to which their home conditions support independent behaviors, and their motivation toward dependent or independent lifestyles before determining their capacity for independent functioning. After these factors have been weighed, an IL program should be devised that provides the training, assistive devices, and psychological support required to attain the highest level of functioning that is both feasible and acceptable to them. When establishing people's optimum levels of functioning, however, care must be taken to distinguish between daily living tasks that are incidental to an independent lifestyle and those that are not. To accomplish this one can use the lifestyles of nondisabled people as a reference point. For example, a married woman who is employed full time and who is not disabled may choose to hire housekeeping help even though it would be possible for her to complete the housekeeping tasks during weekday evenings and weekends. Similarly, a person with a disability who is employed may choose to hire someone to assist with certain tasks, even though he or she may be able to perform these tasks without assistance. In Cappaert's opinion, "If it takes a person forty-five frustrating minutes to accomplish these tasks, while a helper could perform the job in 30 seconds, then it seems absurd to me that the person is often considered to be more independent if they do it themselves" (1979, p. 26).

Often the key to freedom of choice is whether or not an individual has the income necessary to obtain the assistance desired. But certain areas will always exist in which a severely disabled person will have no choice but to rely on someone else. A high-level quadriplegic will have to have someone else mow the lawn, or the lawn will remain unmowed.

What happens, then, to a person who exists on some minimum income assistance program, such as SSI, SSDI, or welfare? Should one's status as a taxpayer or nontaxpayer affect one's ability to choose between a physically independent, and thus less socially burdensome, lifestyle and a physically dependent way of life subsidized by public monies?

Typically, the answer to these questions depends on the person or agency that provides financial support. Workman's Compensation, SSDI, and welfare programs pressure those who can work into working and, increasingly, those who can live outside of institutions into doing so. Only if an individual is financially self-sufficient is he or she allowed true psychological independence, the freedom to live as dependently or independently as he or she chooses. Without documentation that one is physically or mentally incapable of personal and economic self-sufficiency, one is ineligible for most available types of public financial support.

Proponents of the individual-oriented philosophy of independent living, on the one hand, view as a right disability pensions, financial aid to meet the costs of medical treatment, and provision of services that help disabled people compensate for the extraordinary expenses associated with most severely disabling conditions. They believe disabled people are entitled to these benefits because they are members of society and because most contributed to society through productive work and taxes until circumstances beyond their control forced them out of the marketplace. In the case of disabled children, the proponents of the individual-orientation position believe that children's entitlement has been earned through the social contributions of their parents, grandparents, siblings, and other family members.

Proponents of the society-oriented philosophy, on the other hand, view these and similar services as a privilege to be earned, not as a right that automatically accrues to people because they happen to be members of society. From their viewpoint, therefore, recipients must prove that they are worthy of IL services. If potential recipients of services do not prove that the monies spent on them will not be wasted, that they will cooperate with service providers, exercise the skills they learn, and make the best use of the equipment and training they receive, then, these proponents believe, they have forfeited their claim to any support and special consideration.

The society-oriented philosophy reflects the incorporation of people with permanently incapacitating conditions into Parsons' theory (1958) concerning illness and health in our society. What proponents of the individual-oriented philosophy fear is that disabled people will never lose their deviant status, even through increased public awareness of both their needs and their capabilities. They fear that their chances of receiving the adequate medical treatment and social support expected by nondisabled people who are temporarily incapacitated by an accident or acute illness will never be enhanced. They fear that the IL movement will mean that disabled people will be forced to seek out and cooperate with providers of IL services if they wish their existence at a subsistence level to continue to be socially condoned.

## AN INTERMEDIATE PHILOSOPHY
## OF INDEPENDENT LIVING

An intermediate philosophy of independent living, which incorporates both physical and psychological independence to some degree, avoids the problems inherent in orientations that use either physical independence or psychological independence as the criterion that determines the potential and limitations of severely disabled people. This intermediate position assumes that a disability—a physiological condition—is not identical to a handicap—a social condition in which one is unable to perform one or more roles or tasks (see Chapter 1). In reality, many disabled people are conditionally dependent. They may require assistance in self-care or in decision-making or in running a home of their own, but they may still maintain a role as a productive member of society. Many who are incapable of self-care, for example, are remuneratively employed, raise families and work as volunteers within their communities (DeLoach and Greer, 1981; Deyoe, 1972; Laurie, 1977).

For IL services to be maximally effective, the rationale for providing IL services must be expressed in a philosophy that service recipients, as well as service providers, understand and accept. One factor that can enhance or impede the effectiveness of IL services is the motivation of disabled people to live more self-directed lives. Unfortunately, many disabled people are afraid of what they believe are the implications of the IL movement. They fear, as noted above, that nondisabled or less disabled laymen and professionals will expect them to do more for themselves than they are capable of doing. This fear is fostered by those who advocate the society-oriented philosophy. Yet the individual-oriented philosophy also creates problems for the IL movement. If disabled people want to be viewed by others as being just like nondisabled people, in terms of their strengths, their hopes and plans for the future, and their rights as fellow human beings, then advocating the individual-oriented philosophy, in its most extreme form, will be counterproductive. When disabled people demand and expect special treatment that is not related to the specific needs arising from a particular disability, they set themselves apart from, rather than aligning themselves with, the larger society.

A teacher of visually impaired children who is congenitally blind finds that her absence of sight is an asset in helping her students deal realistically with their impairments. She finds that her students, like other children, are expert manipulators, but if they inform her that they are unable to perform an activity because they are "blind," she will know if their blindness is a valid reason or is only being used as an excuse. One question she asks her students regularly to encourage them to risk activities they might otherwise avoid and to analyze how they feel about themselves and their disability is, "What do you think makes you so special?"

Most often it is a person in a helping profession—a teacher, a counselor, an IL specialist—who has both the knowledge and the objectivity to advocate an IL philosophy to and for his or her students or clients that retains the best of the society- and the individual-oriented viewpoints. Such an intermediate philosophy is expressed in the Independent Living Research Utilization Project's definition of independent living as

> control over one's life based on the choice of acceptable options that minimize reliance on others in making decisions and in performing everyday activities. This includes managing one's own affairs; participating in day-to-day life in the community; fulfilling a range of social roles; and making decisions that lead to self-determination and the minimization of psychological or physical dependence on others. Independence is a relative concept, which may be defined personally by each individual. (ILRUP, 1979)

By encouraging self-sufficiency to the degree that is in the best interests of a disabled individual, while at the same time accepting that individual as a full participant in devising, monitoring, and evaluating the results of an individualized IL plan, an IL specialist can effectively promote both optimum physical independence and client control or freedom of choice. With appropriate services, information, and encouragement from helping professionals, disabled people who can never be totally self-sufficient, even in basic self-care activities, will be able to choose the lifestyle they prefer from a number of feasible options, each of which would allow them to maximize their capabilities in some, if not all, areas of their lives.

## INDEPENDENT LIVING FORMATS

Although the concept of independent living is not of recent origin, confusion still exists concerning the similarities and differences among various types of IL programs, centers, and residential centers. In order to facilitate communication among IL service providers and recipients, the Office for Handicapped Research published the following definitions, which were developed by the Independent Living Research Utilization Project in Houston (1979):

> **Independent Living Program** A community-based program which has substantial consumer involvement, provides directly or coordinates indirectly through referral those services necessary to assist severely disabled individuals to increase self-determination and to minimize unnecessary dependence on others.
> Services that must be provided or coordinated are housing provision; attendant, reader and/or interpreter services; and information about goods and services relevant to independent living. Other services that are provided or coordinated by independent living programs include transportation provision or registry, peer counseling, advocacy or political action, independent living skills training, equipment maintenance and repair, and social-recreational services. Note: Custodial care facilities and primary medical care facilities are specifically excluded from the definition of an independent living program. (P. 12)
>
> **Independent Living Service Provider** An organization which provides several discrete services which can be used to increase an individual's opportunities to live independently. While an independent living service provider does not meet the criteria necessary to qualify as an independent living program, the services it provides may be referred to by an independent living program.
>
> **Independent Living Center** A community-based nonprofit, nonresidential program which is controlled by the disabled consumer it serves, provides services directly or coordinates services indirectly

through referral services to assist severely disabled individuals to increase personal self-determination and to minimize unnecessary dependence upon others. The minimum set of services that are provided by an independent living center are housing assistance; attendant, reader and/or interpreter services; peer counseling; financial and legal advocacy; and community awareness and barrier removal programs.

**Independent Living Residential Center**  An independent living program that provides housing, attendant care, and transportation provision or referral. Other services can be provided either as primary or secondary services. (P. 14)

In determining the type of IL program that would best meet the needs of a particular region or community, a variety of factors must be taken into account: the size of the geographical area to be served; the number of people who require services; the types of disabling conditions that predominate; the availability of auxiliary social support services; and, finally, the policy guidelines established by the program's founders or funding agency.

## SIZE OF THE REGION OR COMMUNITY

In heavily populated areas or in areas that draw clients from a wide geographical area, IL services are usually delivered through one or more of four major system designs, although any of a variety of service modes may operate with some success. The first system design consists of a transitional program that provides clients with a variety of services tailored to meet specific needs. The second system design consists of a nonresidential information and referral program that coordinates existing community services and provides some direct services to disabled people who reside in their own homes in the surrounding area. The third system design consists of a long-term residential program that provides additional support services, such as transportation and attendant care. The fourth system design combines features of the first three by providing long-term residential housing, transitional housing, and informational, referral, and direct services (Rice and Roessler, 1980). The New Options program in Houston exemplifies the first of these designs; the Berkeley Center for Independent Living in California (CIL), the second; Timbers, in Wichita, Kansas, the third; and the Boston Center for Independent Living (BCIL), the fourth.

New Options, although located in a populous metropolitan area, is geared toward providing services to clients from other states as well as to those from Texas and the Houston vicinity.

The New Options program, therefore, concentrates on short-term, intensive training of clients in self-care skills, in budget management, or in any other area where they have a functional deficit. In contrast, Berkeley's CIL focuses on long-term services to a sizable and stable group of disabled people residing in the heavily populated Bay Area in California. For example, the CIL-operated wheelchair-accessible vans provide transportation to mobility-impaired people in the seven-city urban area across the bay from San Francisco, and its mobile wheelchair repair unit is available to those who require on-the-spot repairs within the same service area.

## POPULATION OF PEOPLE WITH DISABILITIES

Berkeley's CIL is located in a state with a higher-than-average proportion of disabled people within the 16- to 65-year-old age range (Blake, 1981). While media images may perpetuate the idea that Californians are tanned, lithe models of physical perfection, a 1981 state census revealed that 11.6 percent of all Californians between the ages of 16 and 65, or the normal span of working years, have disabilities that significantly affect their ability to maintain a job (Office of Information and Resources for the Handicapped, 1981). This percentage does not include the 12 percent of children and the 33 percent of elderly people who are disabled and who require special rehabilitation services, but who are outside the age range of those usually considered eligible for traditional vocational rehabilitation services (Blake, 1981; Williams, 1981). Any IL program in California, or a state similar in population and percentage of disabled people, will have a large number of potential clients within a relatively limited area, which will reduce the need for residential facilities.

In states where there are few densely populated urban areas and the people requiring services are scattered over a wide area, uprooting clients from their home communities may not be the most feasible method for providing services. Yet in 1980 only three IL programs that provided services in rural areas had been identified. In rural areas, therefore, services might be facilitated by a mobile IL program. The staff of such a program would move from community to community and work with clients within their homes and general environments. By conducting on-site functional evaluations, consulting directly with clients and families in their homes, and making on-site equipment recommendations and housing modifications, counselors would be in a better position to match client needs with available resources.

PREDOMINANT DISABLING CONDITIONS

The establishment of specific categories of IL services is based on proven need in a particular area. But when establishing IL policies that are designed to meet a community's specific needs, it is also important to consider the region's projected demographic changes, so that policies that meet a community's needs at present are flexible enough to adjust to any changes in the future.

Soon after issue of the regulations for Section 504 (see Chapter 1), which mandated accessibility in programs and buildings supported by government funds, an article appeared in the *Wall Street Journal* concerning a public library in a small rural community. According to the article, there were no mobility-impaired people in the town, and yet the town was threatened with the loss of its library if it wasn't ramped according to the regulations. On the surface, this article made a credible case against a regulation that mandated that buildings be made barrier-free when the proposed modifications would benefit nobody. But what appears to be credible may, upon closer analysis, prove not to be when long-term implications are taken into account. In the case of architectural accessibility, postponement of building modifications can only result in increased modification costs in the future.

Two factors must be considered when the question of barrier-free architecture is broached: (1) building costs will increase over time, and (2) the numbers of people requiring barrier-free facilities will increase over time. At present, 11 percent of the population is over 65, and the total number of people over 65 increases by 1,600 each day. According to the Rehabilitation Services Administration, furthermore, one out of three people over 65 is disabled (Williams, 1981). The reasonableness of regulations that require wheelchair accessibility in the library of a town where no one presently has a mobility impairment becomes apparent when the situation is viewed in terms of future cost-effectiveness (Bowe, 1978). Even if none of the townspeople are amputees or paraplegics, it is in the nature of things that all will age, and disability is a normal component of aging.

Although not all disabled people have impairments that require the use of a walker, crutches, or a wheelchair, many do acquire impairments that make it impossible for them to ascend steps because of excessive energy demands or the dangers of falling as a result of a loss of coordination. With appropriate environmental modifications, elderly disabled people often can continue to live their lives much as they did before they acquired their disabilities (Williams, 1981). Patronizing their community's library is only one of many activities that disabled people of any age can continue to enjoy with minimal accommodation on the part of their communities.

Often a lack of accessible facilities and support services means that providers of IL services must concentrate on an area's current population of disabled people. When establishing programs where no network of support services already exists, organizations or agencies cannot afford to develop services for which there is no present need. Program planners must undertake feasibility studies that investigate which populations are most in need of services as a first step in determining which services should be provided as soon as possible and which can be postponed. Then long-range studies can be conducted to estimate what needs will develop or increase over time. Few communities are as fortunate as the town mentioned above, which, having no citizens in present need of IL services, could utilize resources that it would otherwise expend on existing needs to prepare for those to come.

An often overlooked factor affecting the numbers and types of disabled people who require services is migration. The 1980 U.S. census indicated a general population movement from the Midwest and the Northeast to states in the Sunbelt, triggered, it is believed, by rising energy costs and the economic decline of the former industrial centers of the North. Similarly, populations of disabled people will also shift to areas with climates or terrains more compatible with their functional limitations. Often, when an opportunity for a job transfer arises, families with a disabled family member move to sections of the country where medical and rehabilitation services are concentrated. To a certain extent, it is as true that disabled populations tend to congregate where rehabilitation-related services are already available as that rehabilitation-related services are established to meet the needs of preexisting disabled populations. For example, urban areas near VA hospitals with spinal cord injury units tend to have a high percentage of spinal cord-injured residents who moved to these areas because of the special medical services that were available to them.

It is difficult to determine whether the indigenous incidence of physical limitations is higher in California than elsewhere or if more people with physical limitations live there because of its extensive system of services for disabled persons. With a State Commissioner of Rehabilitation who is a quadriplegic and who has promoted progressive rehabilitation policies on a statewide basis, California has more than 20 IL programs (Seventh Institute on Rehabilitation Issues, 1980). None of the others, however, is as comprehensive as the CIL in Berkeley. California also has a state-wide system of architectural modifications, where the most remote community provides curb-cuts and special parking for disabled people. It would be difficult to estimate the drawing power that the reputation of an established rehabilitation system, such as California's, has on disabled people and their families.

## PRE-EXISTING COMMUNITY SUPPORT SERVICES

The effectiveness of IL programs depends, in part, on the number and kinds of auxiliary support services that already exist in an area. Unless a core of rehabilitation and related services already exists, any single IL program will be hard pressed to provide the range of services the disabled require, such as transportation, housing, income maintenance, and continuing personal and medical care. The fact that many programs are information and referral services that coordinate existing services instead of providing services directly stems from the limitations of having too few staff and financial resources. Even the CIL, which in 1980 had a total budget of 3.5 million dollars, relies on pre-existing community resources. For example, the Center's apartment locator service would be ineffective if accessible apartments did not already exist in the Berkeley area.

The Australian IL system, which is operated as part of the National Health Program, is an outstanding example of a country-wide program that operates effectively within a network of related but auxiliary services. Clients who come to the Australian IL centers, which are primarily clearinghouses for assistive devices, are evaluated, are allowed to take home aids that seem appropriate to their needs, and receive authorization to obtain, without charge, those aids that prove effective (Parameter, 1980). In the Australian system, as in the British Commonwealth, housing, transportation, interpreter aid, mobility training, attendant care, and so on, are the responsibility of service providers other than those who work in the IL centers.

In the United States, in contrast, IL centers and programs are concerned with all aspects of independent living, even when they are unable to provide auxiliary services. The emphasis is on social integration, or "participating in day-to-day life in the community; fulfilling a range of social roles" (ILRUP, 1979). IL programs are given the responsibility for the desired outcome of all independence-related social services, since other service providers often turn to IL programs for information and assistance. Most programs achieve this outcome through the careful coordination and integration of innumerable disparate but interrelated public and private human services.

## FUNDING AND INTRA-AGENCY RESTRICTIONS

What services programs offer is largely determined by the individuals who establish a program or the agencies that fund IL services. Unlike well-established programs, such as New Options or CIL, most fledgling IL programs received their funding under Title VII of the 1978 Amendments to the Rehabilitation Act of 1973. Unlike Part B of Title VII, which does not provide for residential services, Part A has never been funded. Part B, as described in Chapter 1, provides services that are primarily concerned with information and referral, such as housing registries, attendant registries, and so on. If federal funds were made available under Part A, states would have to prove their eligibility for grants by demonstrating that they already have a variety of living arrangements available that provide a reasonable alternative to institutionalization for mentally retarded and disabled people. Part A, therefore, would give states an incentive to provide a variety of direct services that are not now available through programs established under Part B. Among the direct services authorized under Part A would be

> counseling services; including psychological, psychotherapeutic, and related services; housing incidental to the purpose of this section (including appropriate accommodations to and modifications of any space to serve handicapped individuals); appropriate job placement services; transportation; attendant care; physical prostheses and other appliances and devices; health maintenance; recreational activities; services for children of pre-school age, including physical therapy, development of language and communication skills, and child development services; and appropriate preventative services to decrease the needs of individuals assisted under the program for similar services in the future. (Section 701, P.L. 95-602, 1978 Amendments of the 1973 Rehabilitation Act)

Although Part A has never been funded, a variety of modified housing alternatives that have been established through other, usually multiple, funding sources are available. Most residential facilities designed for the severely disabled provide attendant care, along with modified transportation services. Independent living programs, including residential centers that operate on funds from multiple sources, necessarily expend larger proportions of staff time on grant writing and other types of fundraising activities.

The expenditure of staff time and resources to maintain operating monies is compensated for, in part, by the longevity of programs whose existence does not depend on a single funding source. As the cutbacks in government funding for all categories of rehabilitation-related services in 1981 demonstrated, programs that are totally dependent on state and federal monies can be forced to cease operations. While the decrease in available support services was the immediate effect of the 1981 federal budget cuts, the long-term effect was on people in the rehabilitation and related professions and, consequently, on the disabled children and adults they had served. Many in the helping professions were forced out of positions in which they worked with disabled people into positions outside the field of rehabilitation. In addition, people who would otherwise have entered the helping professions were discouraged from committing themselves to careers with uncertain futures. This phenomenon left the disabled not only without desperately needed services but also without the support of some of their most important advocates.

Even though monies continued to be appropriated for programs under Part B of Title VII, programs guidelines did not allow for such needed services as housing modifications, adaptive equipment, or prosthetic devices. Similarly, each supplementary agency had its own guidelines on how grant funds could be expanded. Such guidelines simplify the process of evaluating services and enhance the accountability of service providers. They can, however, complicate attempts to provide services that would enable a severely disabled person to attain and maintain an optimally independent lifestyle.

## FACTORS INFLUENCING INDEPENDENT LIVING GOALS

Once the concept of independent living is accepted as both a humanitarian and a practicable alternative to vocational rehabilitation, the next objective is to efficiently identify the factors that contribute to a severely disabled person's success in achieving maximum independence. After those factors have been identified, rehabilitation professionals can more effectively incorporate them into their work.

### FACTORS AFFECTING CLIENT SUCCESS

Independent living emphasizes the primacy of and the need for control by the client over both the environment and the chosen lifestyle. Independent living is synonymous with client autonomy, but such autonomy is possible only when disabled people are able to control their own affairs and are convinced of their ability to do so. If clients believe that they can live without the supervision of others, even in situations where they remain physically dependent in one or more areas of self-care or living requirements, they will have the confidence to attempt to manage their own lives. The key role of client control or self-governance in IL rehabilitation was recognized by the drafters of the original provisions of the 1978 Amendments. According to this legislation, disabled people are to have an influence on the policies and the operation of all IL programs established with federal funds:

> No grant may be made under this section unless an application therefore has been submitted to and approved by the Commissioner. The Commissioner may not approve an application for a grant unless the application . . . (1) provide assurances that handicapped individuals will be substantially involved in the policy direction and management of such center, and will be employed by such center. . . . (Part B—Centers for Independent Living, Section 711b, [1])

Therefore, the participation of disabled people in the operation of IL programs, through membership in advisory committees, employment as program staff, or involvement as peer counselors, is integral to the underlying service philosophy of such programs. The insistence on participation by disabled people in the policy development, consultation, and day-to-day operation of IL programs is based on the premise that disabled people who themselves are coping with life are more likely to understand the needs of other disabled people and are in a better position to determine how these needs can best be met. For example, peer counseling, a concept that is essential to program success and that has many variations in practice, is based on the assumption that using disabled people as counselors will provide other disabled people with role models who can also serve as personal resources for those who are experiencing difficulties in certain areas. Properly trained and recruited, peer counselors may be able to anticipate questions that might otherwise go unasked, identify problems that might otherwise go undetected, and offer viable alternative solutions to certain living problems that might otherwise overwhelm a newly disabled person or a person who is attempting to live more independently than before.

The significance of the relationship between client autonomy and IL success was demonstrated in a study by Currie-Gross and Heimbach (1980), who discovered that internally oriented (self-directed) subjects displayed greater IL skills in the areas of "mobility, self-care, employment and independent living in general." According to these researchers, independent behaviors seem to be rooted in the conviction that one actually has the ability to manipulate one's environment to a meaningful extent.

## TECHNIQUES AND CONCEPTS
## ESSENTIAL TO SUCCESS

Before IL rehabilitation emerged as a distinct system of social services, the major emphases in rehabilitation were medical rehabilitation (see Chapter 5) and vocational rehabilitation. Medical rehabilitation is concerned primarily with physical restoration, and successful medical rehabilitation is dependent, to a great degree, on the competence of physicians and therapists who perform corrective surgery, strengthen and condition muscles, improve eye-hand coordination, and stabilize basic physiological processes through diet, exercise, and medication. In addition, medical rehabilitation has as an objective the fostering of patients' psychological and social adjustment by helping patients and their families to deal with the fact of disablement and, if necessary, to restructure their lives to accommodate whatever physical and social changes a disability entails.

Vocational rehabilitation builds upon and in its goals is guided by the results of prior medical rehabilitation efforts. The prognoses of medical experts concerning a client's vocational potential determine whether he or she is judged acceptable for vocational rehabilitation services; that is, the criterion is whether he or she will be able to work after receiving appropriate career counseling, training, and placement services. In the past, however, factors outside of medical or vocational rehabilitation's sphere of expertise often contributed to the failure of rehabilitants to fulfill their apparent potential to resume their social roles. Sometimes rehabilitation efforts failed because of a lack of motivation on the rehabilitant's part (see Chapter 13), but often the failure resulted from a lack of other social support services that could not be supplied by medical and rehabilitation professionals.

The ILR concept is not as delimited a set of services as is traditional medical or vocational rehabilitation. By its very nature, ILR is more complex, because it is concerned with the availability and integration of a vast network of direct services that, when combined with information and referral services, can be implemented through a variety of service formats. The global nature of the services that are essential to IL success has been recognized by rehabilitation professionals. According to Walton, Schawb, Cassatt-Dunn, and Wright (1980), when rehabilitation counselors were surveyed to determine what techniques and concepts they believed to be essential to successful IL, they identified the 140 listed in Table 3.1, but stated that 97 of the 140 were not used in the traditional vocational rehabilitation process. Component facets of an independent lifestyle such as sexuality, use of employment services, long-range career development possibilities, use of adaptive or home maintenance equipment, proper use of one's body, information about and help in establishing alternative living accommodations, financing and locating attendant aides, personal budgeting, mode of and adjustments for private transportation, were described as being essential to the successful adjustment of a disabled person to independent living. The services routinely provided to disabled clients do not supply training in any of these areas.

TRAINING AND SKILLS OF IL PERSONNEL

Because of the complexity of IL goals, no one who works as an IL specialist can master all the techniques and concepts identified in the Walton et al. (1980) study. In programs with limited staff, funding and auxiliary services—most typical of small urban and rural areas—essential services, such as those of an occupational therapist who can prescribe and construct assistive devices, must be obtained through contracts for parttime services. In large urban areas, an IL program may include a variety of rehabilitation specialists, including a fulltime occupational therapist or rehabilitation engineer, among its staff.

From a service provider's point of view, the process of first establishing and then working to attain the goals set for individual clients is costly in staff time and program resources (Rice and Roessler, 1980). The complex, individualized nature of the required services often means that procedures and devices that ensure success for one client will bear little or no resemblance to procedures or devices that ensure success for another. In situations like Ernie's (see Chapters 2 and 9), where the potential for complete independence in everyday activities exists, most of the techniques and concepts identified in Table 3.1 may have to be considered for optimum success. In a situation like Eleanor's, however, clients who are older will have already mastered many basic living skills that will not be affected by the disability, for example, general money management. People like Eleanor, however, may require supplementary budgetary training specific to

TABLE 3.1 TECHNIQUES AND CONCEPTS FOUND TO BE SIGNIFICANT TO INDEPENDENT LIVING

PERSONAL ADJUSTMENT

**Adjustment to Disability**
Realization and evaluation of personal and family roles
Development of assertive behaviors
Utilization of unstructured time
Development of a sense of responsibility
Sense of self-esteem

**Decision-Making with Relationship to Problem-Solving**
Problem identification
Process of thinking through problem
Application of solution to problem
Evaluation of alternative solutions

DOMESTIC ARRANGEMENTS

**Home Maintenance***
Realistic standards for housekeeping
Use/adaptability of housekeeping equipment
Use of vacuum cleaner
Use of washer/dryer
Use/adaptability of home-maintenance equipment
Selection of equipment
Selection of utensils, appliances
Equipment durability, versatility
Ease of use, cleaning equipment
Equipment safety features
Equipment guarantees, warranties
Types of controls on equipment
Changing order of tasks
Arranging workspace

**Food Preparation***
Meal planning
Selection of food in stores
Techniques for food preparation
Convenience food cooking
Equipment and technique for dishwashing
Use and adaptability of electrical equipment
Use of electric can opener
Use of hand-held mixer
Use of electric skillet
Use of toasters
Use of refrigerators
Use of range/oven
Use of coffee pots
Use/adaptability of manual kitchen equipment

Use of surface burner
Use of utensils
Basic nutrition

MANAGEMENT SKILLS

**Self-Management***
Personal care: upkeep of appearance
Clothing selection for protection and safety
Clothing features to look for in ready-to-wear clothing
Clothing care
Clothing selection for easy on and off
Physical care
Knowledge of the etiology and progression of disability
Self-controlled medical maintenance procedures
Recognition of need for changes in medication
Identification of personal range of motion
Analysis of personal techniques to take advantage of mobility
Development of emergency care
Financing attendant/aids
Locating attendant/aids
Transfer techniques
Modes of and adjustments for private transportation

**Child Care***
Physical care of child
Child playtime activities, supervision
Care and selection of children's clothing, equipment, and furniture
Emotional and motor, language and social growth

**Financial Management***
Awareness of programs of financial assistance
Using bank accounts
Personal budgeting
Making change
Using credit
Investments, insurance, long-term planning
Discounts for elderly and disabled people

**Time Management***
Application of time analysis in time scheduling

*(continued)*

**TABLE 3.1,** *continued*

Application of time analysis in time planning
Utilization of time in purposeful activity

SOCIAL ADJUSTMENT
**With Family**
Family member roles
Family activities
Family decision-making
Inclusion of entire family in the rehabilitation process

**With Others**
Development of communication skills
Interpretation of verbal and body language
Getting along with other people
Ability to initiate and maintain personally and mutually satisfying relationships
Recognition and acceptance of one's effect on others
Sense of loving and caring for another person
Right to privacy
Management of ongoing relationships

**Sexuality: Recognition of Role Expectations***
Self-understanding
Analysis and acceptance of role expectations of significant others
The dating process
Physical aspects of sexuality
Awareness of family planning alternatives
Knowledge of and education for sexual expression
Alternatives
Awareness of changing sexual relationships
Knowledge of sexual aids and devices

**Leisure Time***
Recognition/application of abilities that can be used to develop and/or participate in activities
Games suited to specific needs/likes/interests
Hobbies suited to specific needs/likes/interests

**Identification and Utilization of Community Support Services**
Awareness of community government
Retailers in community with special services available to disabled people
Manufacturers producing products designed for special needs
Current literature
Awareness of medical resources in the community
Special interest groups dealing with disability
Awareness of private agencies
Analysis of services provided for special needs
Awareness of special interest groups
Educational or vocational services, schools, or facilities
Techniques in group counseling
Community services that can aid in solutions

**Knowledge of the World of Work***
Development of use of employment/placement services
Initiation of specific referrals
Awareness of entry-level requirements
Career development possibilities
Level of income
Taxation responsibilities
Self-perception as a worker

**Housing Arrangements***
Alternative living situations other than family
Services available to organize and conduct alternative living
House planning and remodeling
Kitchen arrangements and adaptations
Entrances/doors
Ramps
Bathrooms (accessibility)
Laundry facilities/procedures
Housekeeping supplies, safety and use
Housecleaning adaptive procedures
Housecleaning adaptive equipment
Awareness of professional services
Storage principles
Analysis of task necessity

*(continued)*

**TABLE 3.1,** *continued*

| Transportation Arrangements | Miscellaneous |
| --- | --- |
| Aids that can be used to increase ease of transportation | Individual and/or family rehabilitation counseling |
| Modes of public and private transportation | Available psychological care |
| | Utilization of team approach in meeting IL needs |

*Techniques and concepts not typically utilized by vocational rehabilitation counselors as part of their jobs (Walton et al., 1980, pp. 59–63).

their situation, such as how to negotiate for a lower price on medications purchased in large quantities (Bruck, 1978). For Eleanor, aspects of training requiring emphasis might include self-care and household management or how best to acquire and retain help from others in carrying out these tasks. Because of her age and the likelihood of additional physical limitations, Eleanor should be counseled about the proper use of her body, especially those joints likely to be affected by the osteoarthritic process.

For Ernie, the emphasis in IL services would be on the development of emotional and financial resources because of his potential ability to establish a home and family of his own. In view of his youth and lack of any secondary disabilities, rehabilitative success might depend upon Ernie's continuing to maintain his psychological and financial independence for several decades. Since Eleanor is in a more precarious situation, physically, success might be determined by how long she remains at her present level of independent functioning, before her arthritic condition progresses to the point where she has a renewed need for IL services.

In every case IL personnel must address the client's immediate IL concerns, using techniques designed to moderate any decrease in ability to function. An independent living program (ILP) (see Chapters 1 and 9) designed to meet Ernie's needs would provide him with an opportunity to relearn and practice self-care skills learned during his medical rehabilitation. Additional training could be provided in home management and in preparing for a suitable vocation. Among the techniques and concepts appropriate in Ernie's case would be referral to accessible housing sites, adaptation of the home he chooses, training in budget management, access to traditional VR services, and peer counseling in the areas of sexuality and family relations. Independent living services for Eleanor would include interim housekeeping services, transportation, temporary attendant care, and training in self-care and homemaking techniques geared to her diminishing physical capacities.

Educational programs that are designed to train IL counselors can build on fundamental rehabilitation techniques and concepts already included in traditional counselor education programs. Under IL guidelines, however, such programs would expand their traditional emphasis on knowledge of and ability to integrate existing community resources. They would continue to foster the counseling and managerial skills of counselors-in-training, while adding rehabilitation-related subjects, such as counseling for people with emotional, mental and physical disabilities, that have been missing in or incidental to rehabilitation counseling programs (Roessler, 1981).

In an article entitled "Development of an Independent Living Program Curriculum," Geist (1980) compiled a list of competency areas required by IL personnel that included

> advocacy skills, technology utilization in both biomechanics and job engineering, assertiveness training and communication skills, sexuality for the disabled and socialization skills, more inclusive activities of daily living using community resources, incentives and disincentives to an independent life style, transportation issues, attendant care and management of personnel, use of peer counselors, knowing where the rehabilitation counselor fits into the process of ILR, and the attitudes and philosophical basis for non-vocational goals. (P. 54)

Geist also interviewed directors of IL programs to determine whether they saw a need for rehabilitation counselors as IL staff members and, where they saw such a need, what skills they thought these counselors should possess. Although those interviewed stated that rehabilitation counselors were needed in IL programs, Geist concluded that their response was influenced by the fact that at the time of the survey there were no other professional groups with the broad background and training needed to achieve global IL goals. According to Geist, other rehabilitation-related professionals are more specialized, and so have a more limited view of the nature and goals of independent living. While their area of specialization makes certain professionals, such as occupational therapists, invaluable in solving specific IL problems, their high degree of specialization also renders them less able to understand and help disabled persons meet the myriad demands that leading an independent lifestyle entails.

In keeping with the wide-ranging nature of program services, therefore, the directors of IL programs emphasized the importance of an indepth knowledge of the psychosocial effects of disabling conditions. Other areas of competence that program directors identified as essential in enhancing clients' IL success were good counseling and good communication skills, especially in the areas of sexuality and assertiveness training.

Paradoxically, while sexuality, assertiveness training, and psychosocial aspects of disabling conditions are already in the core curricula of accredited rehabilitation counselor training programs, these are the areas that state agency directors believe are least important in their counselors' work with vocational rehabilitation clients (Rubin and Roessler, 1978). According to Rubin and Roessler, counselors in state agencies not only get little recognition for their competencies in these areas, but are often actively forbidden to exercise their counseling skills or use their knowledge of the psychosocial aspects of disabling conditions. Research indicates, however, that from the working counselor's point of view, the skills developed in counselor education programs, as defined by the accrediting body, the Council on Rehabilitation Education (CORE), are as suited to the needs of independent living rehabilitation as to the needs of vocational rehabilitation. Furthermore, these counseling skills have been described as more rewarding to exercise than the case management, supervisory, and clerical skills that state agency counselors practice most of the time (Rubin and Roessler, 1978).

# 4

## Independent Living:
## A Combination of Cost-Effectiveness
## and Humanitarian Principles

Perhaps one of the most important things that can be done to support a newly emerging area of human service is to systematically develop a sound rationale for the new service effort. The professionals and the clients of the service area are likely to be the only people who understand and appreciate the impact the new service effort can have upon the lives of people in need. Much of the opposition to implementing new programs comes from people who simply do not know what legitimate contributions these programs can make. The best way to prevent and overcome that opposition is for those who do understand the new service effort—that is, clients and professionals—to educate those who do not.

At a recent social gathering, a gentleman was discussing special education services with one of the authors. He said that he was distressed to hear about teachers in public schools having to give an inordinate amount of time and attention to students in hospital beds who were being mainstreamed into the public school system. He went on to say that he thought such practices were unfair to nonhandicapped children in that teachers did not have enough time to spend with them after taking care of the "bedridden" students.

Apparently this gentleman had been the unfortunate recipient of false and incomplete information regarding mainstreaming, yet he had believed and was disturbed about what he had heard. This man is not uneducated, nor is he simply out of touch with the world. In fact, he is a successful university professor, a writer, and a consultant. He enjoys a handsome income and has considerable influence in his community, his home state, and his profession. The fact that such a person can be so completely misled underscores the need to develop a sound rationale for all new service programs and to inform the public about them. Independent living services are certainly no exception to this rule.

In discussing the rationale or philosophical basis for a public service program it is necessary to address two questions. First, should the specific service under consideration be provided? If the answer is "yes," then a second question arises: What is the most effective and efficient way to provide the service?

This chapter will deal with the first question only. Should IL services be provided to disabled and elderly citizens? Rubin and Roessler's (1978) discussion of the philosophical justification for vocational rehabilitation services provides a format useful in addressing this question. First, the justification for IL services will be discussed from an economic perspective. Then a justification from a purely humanitarian perspective will be discussed. The positive and negative implications of each position will be considered. Finally, a justification will be presented that integrates the most positive aspects of both these positions.

## THE ECONOMIC ARGUMENT

The first argument in support of independent living services is an economic one. Many, if not all, proponents of community-based IL service agencies argue that such programs are a more cost-effective way of meeting the needs of severely disabled and elderly people than the more traditional methods of nursing homes or other total care institutions. It is claimed that IL services are a wise investment of funds in at least three ways. Each of these is discussed briefly.

### COSTS PER CLIENT PER YEAR

The cost of serving a severely disabled or older person in a community-based program designed to enhance the ability of its clients to live independently is much less than the cost of serving that person in a total care facility. For example, Howse (1980) reports the average cost for institutional care in New York City to be $29,000 per client per year, and Provencal (1980, p. 40) reports that institutional cost per client in Michigan "averages from $55 a day," or over $20,000 per year. On the other hand, these same authors report, community-based service programs are less expensive by one-half, and in some cases even more. Data reported by other authors (see Heal, Sigelman, and Switzky, 1980) also confirm that total care institutions seem to cost about twice as much per client per year as community-based service programs.

A word of caution must be added regarding cost comparisons. Heal et al. (1980) report that adequate data for such comparison purposes have not yet been compiled. The cost figures reported by the various agencies involved often do not report comparable data. The costs of buildings and permanent furnishings may be included in some reports and not in others, and the same is true for other important costs such as program services. As long as such disparities in reporting exist, it will be difficult to assess accurately the comparative costs of community-based and institutional programs.

## SHORT-TERM VERSUS LONG-TERM COSTS

Independent living services may also be a wise investment in terms of long-term costs. The key notion here is preventive treatment.

In recent years insurance companies have increasingly turned toward preventive treatment as a means of reducing their long-term costs. In the case of a person who is quadriplegic and who is covered by some insurance benefit such as long-term disability or workers' compensation insurance, it is a wise investment of funds to provide top-quality medical care and related services in order to enable the person to live independently at home. Such services may be very expensive in the short run, but they may save the insurance company much more than they cost over a long period of time. The reason for the savings is obvious. A person who is quadriplegic and receives adequate services will probably live at home with minimal, relatively low-cost assistance. On the other hand, if that person does not receive proper care and training in living independently he could be repeatedly hospitalized for pressure sores or other complications, and could require health care services that would be enormous in cost. The insurance company would indeed be foolish not to provide the services needed to prevent such long-term problems, and their provision is becoming the trend in the industry.

This same argument holds true in government-funded human service agencies. The long-term costs of not providing adequate services to newly disabled and elderly people may well be much more than the costs of those services themselves. For example, Eleanor, one of the case studies discussed in Chapter 2, had to resort to living in a nursing home after her surgery because no one had arranged support services that would enable her to live at home. The costs to society of that nursing home were much higher than the cost of providing the necessary support services for Eleanor to live at home would have been. When she later returned home after making arrangements for support services herself, she was much happier, and the cost of her supportive services were strikingly lower than the nursing home costs. Thus the net long-run savings gained by providing high-quality IL services provide another example of its sound economic justification.

## SERVICES THAT RESULT IN EMPLOYABILITY

One might think that services that result in a person becoming employable are confined to the vocational rehabilitation area, but that is not always the case. Often IL services make a valuable contribution to the employability of a disabled person or some member of that person's family. For example, a severely disabled person who is living in a total care institution is certainly not likely to be employed. The reasons that he or she is not employed, however, may depend on such factors as lack of mobility and transportation to and from work, remoteness and isolation of the facility from areas where work is more readily available, and similar problems that might be overcome in a different living environment. If that disabled individual were moved into a community living environment, assisted by proper attendant care, and provided with accessible transportation, he or she might then be a realistic candidate for employment—a fact demonstrated by many successfully employed severely disabled people.

Another contribution to employment made by IL services is in enabling family members to work. A severely disabled person who requires a great deal of assistance may place such demands for attendant services upon some family member that that person is not able to maintain a job. IL services could perhaps reduce the disabled person's need for attendant care, and help to provide the attendant care that is needed. The family member, thus, would be free to hold a full-time job.

In both of the cases described above, the economic gains are that a person is working and paying taxes who otherwise would not be. In addition, that person is less likely to be dependent upon some form of income supplement from the government. Finally, the fact that the person is working, earning money, and spending money is a stimulus to the economy in general.

The justification of IL services from an economic perspective is based on the three preceding arguments. Such services are said to be less expensive on a cost per client per year basis; they reduce long-term costs; and they sometimes enable either the disabled person or a family member to work, produce economically, and pay taxes. Does this mean that advocating IL services as an economically sound measure is the best way to ensure support for this service model? That question will now be addressed by outlining both the positive and negative implications of this argument.

POSITIVE IMPLICATIONS

As one can see by reviewing the economic position, there are some very persuasive figures suggesting that IL is indeed a cost-effective service paradigm. This type of information is generally viewed very positively by people in this society, including those who hold elected offices, and thus this argument has a strong appeal. As long as empirical data suggest that IL services are, in effect, saving money for the taxpayer then this rationale for supporting this program should have favorable results.

A second positive implication of this supporting rationale is that it can be used to encourage worker efficiency. A frequent criticism of government programs is that there is an inexcusable amount of worker inefficiency, waste, and even fraud. If a program such as IL is based upon the underlying premise that it will save money, and if workers in that program are made aware of that premise and are reminded of it from time to time, then one might reasonably expect that the effect on the workers will be to cause them to try to serve all their clients in ways that are as cost-effective as possible. In other words, the underlying rationale for the existence of the program would be made an integral part of the daily work of the employees. The net result would be a program as free as possible of the waste so often criticized in government-operated programs.

The third positive implication of this position is that it provides the opportunity for objective accountability measures based upon hard data. One of the most awkward problems of government-operated human service programs is their inability to point to objective measures of successful operation. It is very difficult to measure the degree to which the quality of life of a group of people has benefited by a government services program. It is much easier, however, to measure the cost of meeting needs through IL programs rather than through other service models, and it is quite satisfying to see in one's hand the reports that indicate that the program one has supported is paying off. That kind of satisfaction is often denied those who are looking for the more elusive evidence of a program's impact upon the quality of the daily life of its clients.

NEGATIVE IMPLICATIONS

To justify the existence of IL service programs on the basis of an economic argument is not without its hazards. The first problem with this justification is that it leaves the program very vulnerable to total abandonment if it ceases to produce data indicating that it is indeed operating in a cost-effective manner. In other words, if the program is sold on the premise that it is more cost-effective, then one cannot expect continued support if it becomes less cost-effective than some other option.

Related to this is the fact that the cost-effectiveness of IL services, as of any service program, can be adversely affected by a number of variables beyond the control of the program staff. Inflation can increase costs, at times, at rates faster than even the best administrator would have estimated. Supporting agencies can make decisions that drive up costs for the IL service program. In one Southern city, for example, a newly established IL service program is having to deal with a crisis in the mass transit system. That entire system is in financial trouble. If it goes out of business, as appears possible, then the costs of transportation services for the clients of the new IL program will skyrocket. That eventuality is completely beyond the control of the IL program staff, yet it could seriously affect the cost-effectiveness of their program.

A third problem is that cost-effectiveness does not mean that the total costs of serving elderly and severely disabled people will immediately decrease. As Howse (1980) points out, established total care institutions are not going to be closed immediately after community-based IL programs are established. Those institutions will still be needed to serve a small segment of the population for whom no other current option is feasible. In time, perhaps, some of these institutions can be closed and others more effectively used to serve an appropriate clientele. In the meantime the result of maintaining these institutions while developing more cost-effective, community-based programs will be that the total resources devoted to this area of human services will need to be increased.

A fourth difficulty with the economic argument is that it fails to recognize that in some cases costs are not so much reduced as simply transferred to the family. In some cases of deinstitutionalization, an individual is removed from an institution and returned home to live with his or her family. There may be less cost to the state for the maintenance and housing of that person, but that cost is being paid by the family. This is not universally true, but it is true in some cases.

Under the positive implications of this argument it was suggested that this program rationale can be used to enhance worker efficiency. Unfortunately, it might just as easily contribute to a counterproductive attitude. Program workers could become so interested in saving money and making sure that the IL program pays off that they become selective in choosing clients. They may discourage those clients who, they believe, have little potential for success and concentrate their efforts on those they think will produce the highest success rates. This type of attitude could permeate the entire staff of an IL program, and thus cause it to leave unserved those most in need of its services.

Finally, basing the justification for an IL program on economic grounds could contribute to serious problems when clients and workers disagree about what constitutes an appropriate plan of action. If a professional team of workers believes that a particular client is capable of and ready for independent life in the community, but the client believes that he needs the more restrictive, expensive, yet supportive services of a total care institution, then the team members have a very difficult problem. Should they push their client out of the nest and force him to fly on his own, or should they allow him to choose freely the service program he wants? An economic program rationale might encourage the team to pressure the client into choosing the less expensive service option since, in their professional judgment, it is within his capacity. This is a situation in which few professionals want to find themselves. It also is a situation that seems to belie one of the most basic goals of IL service programs: to enable disabled people to make basic life decisions for themselves.

## THE HUMANITARIAN ARGUMENT

With all the factors involved, the economic rationale just described is a complex argument. By contrast, the humanitarian argument is quite simple. In the opinion of some who support the concept of IL services on the basis of humanitarian principles, there is hardly a need even to discuss the rationale for providing such services. They would say that the justification for IL services is self-evident.

Many people are now living completely dependent lives as a result of their disability or their age. They are living with over-protective families, in institutions, and in total care nursing homes. In any of these situations it is all too likely that the restrictions on their opportunities to exercise their functional abilities will cause those abilities to degenerate even further, and therefore their chances of improving enough to be able to move into the community to live independently are practically nil. In their current situations, these people do not have the freedom to choose their own lifestyle and to make their own decisions, a freedom that is characteristic of adults in this society. The final result is that they are relegated to lives of excessive restriction and second-class citizenship.

Given the circumstances just described, many proponents of IL services argue, the provision of these services is a simple and clear-cut value decision. The people of this society "should" pro-vide IL services because they will result in a higher quality of life for the disabled and elderly citizen. These programs will enhance the dignity of their clients, and that is reason enough to provide them. This position is simply a moral or a value judgment.

As before, this argument has positive and negative implica-tions.

## POSITIVE IMPLICATIONS

As mentioned earlier the humanitarian argument is quite simple compared to the economic argument. That simplicity is one of its advantages. In using it to seek support for IL services, one does not have to deal as much with complex questions of costs and benefits. One simply appeals to the conscience of the public and of legislative bodies.

Another positive implication of this argument is that its under-lying premise is not affected by the vicissitudes of cost factors. When making value decisions, people do not usually consider the costs of an action as much as its "rightness." This argument pre-sents IL services as the right response to the needs of severely disabled and elderly people regardless of what the costs might be. The economic insensitivity of this argument is particularly advan-tageous in an era of difficult economic problems and severe bud-get cuts.

## NEGATIVE IMPLICATIONS

The first negative implication of the humanitarian argument is simply the "flip-side" of one of its positive implications. It was stated earlier that this argument posits IL services as the right approach to severely disabled and elderly people's needs, regardless of costs. That is an advantage only so long as people generally share that opinion. Unfortunately, this society is often directed more by economic issues than by humanitarian principles. It often happens that the legislative and governmental bodies of this society respond to difficult economic problems with severe restrictions in spending for social programs. The attitude demonstrated in such times seems to be that, regardless of their humanitarian benefits, these social programs simply cost more than this society can afford. That, of course, is exactly the opposite of the basic premise of the humanitarian position, but nevertheless it seems to be a reality with which IL programs must cope.

The second negative implication of this justification for IL services is that accountability is difficult for such a program. In recent years government agencies have been under increasing pressure to demonstrate that their programs are effective. In the area of human services, that is often a difficult task. If one claims that a specific program's goal is to increase quality of life, personal independence, or some similar goal, then one must be ready and able to clarify the meaning of that goal in terms that are clear and measurable. Thus, accountability becomes a matter of specifying goals in very precise terms, documenting the attainment of those goals by the program and its clients, and documenting the contribution made by the program's services to the attainment of client goals. This process is difficult, time-consuming, and even at best it never seems to adequately state the really valuable contributions of the program. At its worst, it becomes itself the real goal and overriding concern of the program staff, while important client services take second priority and become merely the means by which the staff can compile an impressive accountability record.

The third negative implication of the humanitarian position is the problem that arises when one attempts to define such concepts as "higher quality" or "less restrictive." The staff of IL programs may be convinced that their purpose in serving their clients is to help them attain greater independence and higher quality lives. However, it is certainly possible that some clients of IL programs may disagree as to what constitutes "higher quality." For example, it was noted in Chapter 2 that Marie S. does not want to leave the developmental center to receive services in a community-based program that should lead to a higher quality life than she now has. From an outsider's perspective, such as that of the center's assistant director, the community-based option would definitely lead to a higher quality life, and would even be less expensive, yet Marie does not perceive that option as preferable. She would rather stay where she is than risk the unknown life outside the institution. In such a case as this the perceived purpose of the IL services program staff is thwarted by the client's perception of higher quality.

## INDEPENDENT LIVING: A BETTER BARGAIN

Most often the justification for human service programs is based on either their humanitarian contributions or their economic costs and benefits. It is clear that neither justification is free of disadvantages. Because of these disadvantages, an alternative justification is suggested here. This justification is based on the positive aspects of both the economic and humanitarian arguments. Simply put, it states that even though a lot of money and effort is now being spent on traditional, institutionally based service programs for disabled and elderly people, the most desirable objectives in the lives of these people are not being achieved. The IL service paradigm would more nearly achieve those objectives. Thus, it constitutes a better bargain for the money and effort expended.

To clarify this argument, consider again the case of Marie S. As already noted, it costs a lot of money to keep Marie, and other people with similar problems, in the developmental center. Yet Marie is still restricted, isolated, dependent, unable to make her own decisions about basic life issues, and otherwise subjected to the second-class citizenship of institutional life. In other words, a lot of money and effort is being expended and less than desirable results are being achieved.

If, on the other hand, Marie were to move into the community-based group home mentioned earlier, she would be encouraged and taught to begin to involve herself in her community, to learn to care for her own needs, to make her own decisions as much as possible, and to claim her rights as a fully equal human being in her society. Her personal independence and her quality of life, as measured by the norms of her society, would indeed be enhanced.

To offer the option of the community-based group home while continuing to maintain and operate the developmental center means that more money must be allocated to this area of human need. Yet this additional commitment of resources seems more than worthwhile. Without it people like Marie are being served in ways that are very expensive, yet are relatively ineffective in helping people to become less dependent upon supportive services. In this sense IL services are a real bargain. They more nearly achieve what most human service agencies would like to achieve with their client: personal independence. They also happen to achieve that goal at a cost per client that is considerably lower than that for institutional care.

In the final analysis, this seems to be the most potent justification for IL services. It is effective in achieving its stated objectives, and at the same time it is also cost-effective. But more than that, it accomplishes that most important objective, personal independence, more fully than any other service paradigm.

# PART TWO

*Essential Support Services*

# 5

## Medical Rehabilitation: Foundation for Independent Living Rehabilitation

The term "medical rehabilitation" may have vastly different connotations for laymen and rehabilitation professionals. To some, medical rehabilitation implies failure. In their view the fact that rehabilitation services are required indicates that someone is physically impaired to some degree. They believe, further, not only that people with physical impairments—that is, disabilities—must restructure their entire lives, but also that they must live less satisfying, less productive lives as a result.

In the view of others, medical rehabilitation implies success. To them medical rehabilitation provides treatment and assistive aids and devices that allow visually impaired people to "see" well enough to function on a par with those with no visual impairments, people with damaged hearts to continue to lead active, fulfilling lives, and people with mobility impairments to move about freely in appropriately modified environments. To them, medical rehabilitation professionals perform miracles on a daily basis and help transform disabled people into people who happen to have disabilities but who continue to lead productive, satisfying lives. They know, because of their personal or professional experiences, that medical rehabilitation, through drugs, surgical techniques, functional training, and assistive devices, is able to transform many of those with disabilities into people who are not handicapped by their physical impairments.

This chapter will

1. define and describe the goals of medical rehabilitation,

2. describe the settings in which medical rehabilitation services are offered,

3. explain the stages of the medical rehabilitation process and relate those stages to the progress of people with traumatic or degenerative disabilities,

4. discuss the disincentives to independent lifestyles that stem from traditional medical rehabilitation policies.

## GOALS OF MEDICAL REHABILITATION

When their basic components are identified, all definitions of medical rehabilitation relate the art and science of medicine to the physical, psychological, and social amelioration of the circumstances of disabled people (Hirschberg, Lewis, and Vaughn, 1976; Hylbert and Hylbert, 1979; Rusk, 1977). In theory, then, medical rehabilitation gives equal emphasis to the physical and the psychosocial aspects of disabling conditions. In practice, however, physical restoration is the first priority (Kutner, 1971).

According to Kutner, the emphasis of medical rehabilitation on physical restoration is based on the reasoning that when physical restoration is successful, psychological and social advantages will automatically follow. Unfortunately, as Kutner points out, this reasoning leads to medical rehabilitation policies that neglect procedures that could result in more severely disabled people resuming their chosen social and vocational roles. Moreover, the assumption that physical restoration is a necessary prerequisite for successful role resumption implies that when physical restoration efforts are unsuccessful, full role restoration is impossible.

Because this assumption is unfounded, the inferior status of psychosocial concerns within the medical model of treatment has been criticized from within the medical profession itself (Berman, 1978; Kutner, 1971; Stein, 1978). As Kutner and others have pointed out, when psychosocial concerns, especially those of newly disabled people, are neglected within the medical treatment process, disabled people tend to have more difficulty coping with life outside of medical or custodial settings than their actual physical limitations warrant. What is more, their reduced ability to cope may persist throughout their lives, unless they receive psychological support and training in social skills as anciliary rehabilitation services that, like those offered by IL programs, augment the services received in the medical rehabilitation process.

## MEDICAL REHABILITATION SETTINGS

Whether a medical rehabilitation program gives equal emphasis to physical and psychosocial concerns or limits itself to the goal of physical restoration depends largely on the setting in which the program is carried out. The four typical settings in which medical rehabilitation services are offered are (1) a general medical hospital that offers limited medical rehabilitation services and has no clearly designated area as a site for physical medicine and rehabilitation services; (2) a general medical hospital that has a physical medicine and rehabilitation service that is clearly designated by site and function; (3) a general medical hospital that has a separate wing or building where medical rehabilitation services are located; and (4) a comprehensive medical rehabilitation center that has complete on-site medical services, that may or may not be linked administratively with a medical center complex, and that operates autonomously in the day-to-day treatment of disabled people.

### LIMITED AND DIFFUSE MEDICAL REHABILITATION SERVICES

In most general medical hospital settings, medical rehabilitation services are limited. A patient who is confined to bed for an extended period of time may receive physical therapy once or twice a day from a therapist who exercises the patient in bed. Such passive exercises, where the patient lies quietly while someone else moves his limbs for him, help to keep muscles from atrophying and joint contractures from developing. Although limited, such services are valuable in that they prevent disabling conditions that might otherwise result as a consequence of prolonged hospitalization.

For example, Sally J. was transferred from a general medical hospital to a comprehensive medical rehabilitation center in

Warm Springs, Georgia, following a long illness that involved a high fever and severe abdominal pain. During the weeks that her illness was being diagnosed, Sally had lain with her legs drawn up to her chest for so long that she had developed flexion contractures of her hips and knees. She would not have needed rehabilitation services for the contractures if she had had physical therapy to prevent the consequences of inappropriate positioning in bed.

Limited and diffuse medical rehabilitation services, although useful in preventing conditions like Sally's from developing, are not effective in the medical rehabilitation of chronically ill or disabled people. When Eleanor M. (see Chapter 2) had her corrective hip surgery, she was hospitalized in a setting with limited medical rehabilitation services. Although she received physical therapy, first in the form of passive bed exercises and later in the form of standing exercises and gait training, she did not receive the kind of medical rehabilitation services that might have allowed her to avoid being transferred to the nursing home where her physical condition deteriorated. In communities where only limited medical rehabilitation services are available, IL programs that coordinate and provide services such as housing, attendant care, physical and occupational therapy, and transportation, are even more important than they are in communities where these services are available through existing medical rehabilitation settings.

## CENTRALLY LOCATED SERVICES
## IN GENERAL MEDICAL HOSPITALS

When a general medical hospital has a distinct area that is clearly identified as the area where medical rehabilitation services originate, it usually has more than one category of medical rehabilitation professional on its staff. According to Hirschberg et al., the most limited of these centralized medical rehabilitation settings will have, in addition to a physician and a nurse, a rehabilitation therapist and a social worker.

Such settings, however, because of their limited staff and physical facilities, will not be able to effectively meet the medical rehabilitation needs of severely disabled people. Although those who acquire severe physical disabilities may receive adequate acute medical treatment in these settings, they will have to be transferred eventually to more comprehensive medical rehabilitation settings if they are to attain an optimum level of functional ability.

## ANNEXED OR CENTRALLY LOCATED
## IN-HOUSE SETTINGS

The third type of medical rehabilitation setting is one in which the site of medical rehabilitation services is physically separate from but still functionally part of a larger, general medical hospital or medical center. Medical rehabilitation services that are housed separately have a distinct advantage over those physically incorporated into a general medical hospital. First, because their operational needs, from cleaning to nursing, are distinct, separately housed settings have large staffs that represent most of the rehabilitation professions. Second, in these settings every staff member, from custodian to medical resident, can more easily be oriented toward medical rehabilitation goals. The very ambience of a medical rehabilitation setting that is physically remote from the area where acutely or terminally ill persons are being treated is more conducive to rehabilitation success than are settings where physically disabled people are viewed as sick patients, rather than as physically well people who need training as much as treatment to alleviate the effects of their disabling conditions.

Separately housed medical rehabilitation settings, in addition to their emphasis on physical restoration, also tend to give a high priority to role restoration. Although therapy schedules are still established and strictly maintained, these settings foster self-directed behaviors on the part of their disabled residents/patients more than do general medical settings. Since residents/patients are not, and are not considered to be, acutely ill, they are allowed greater freedom in the way they dress, spend their free time, and arrange the quarters in which they live. People who are receiving medical rehabilitation services in these settings are expected to wear street clothes during the day, to go to bed at night when they choose, and to independently explore the rehabilitation facility's grounds and the surrounding community. Autonomous behaviors are encouraged at all times, except when they interfere with prescribed therapy schedules. Regardless of how progressive a medical rehabilitation setting's philosophy of treatment is, the overall goals of treatment depend on adherence to carefully planned and designed therapeutic regimens.

To a visitor the most noticeable difference in separately housed settings is that the residents/patients are often indistinguishable from the staff. For example, at Craig, patients and staff dress in casual street clothes. Since some staff members are themselves severely physically disabled, with no uniforms to distinguish them from the people with whom they work, an outsider is forced to treat everyone with the respect that is often only accorded the rehabilitation staff (Kerr, 1972). Simple policy adjustments, such as having staff members dress in the same manner as the residents/patients, can have a great effect on the way that disabled people are viewed and treated and on how they feel about themselves (Kerr, 1972).

## COMPREHENSIVE MEDICAL REHABILITATION SETTINGS

Comprehensive medical rehabilitation settings provide services that are designed to increase disabled people's ability to function, physically and socially. In such settings the myth that people with physical limitations must also be limited psychologically—in their ability to make decisions and manage their own lives—is more easily dispelled, because professionals in such settings work with people who are not acutely ill. Any prescribed medical treatment, therefore, is to maintain, control, or improve their physical function. Moreover, a great deal of the rehabilitation regimen is aimed at improving their ability to cope with the demands of daily living, both physical and psychological.

Comprehensive medical rehabilitation settings are designed to utilize general medical resources that exist within the surrounding community but seldom have a direct affiliation with another hospital. Unlike the settings described above, these settings are comprehensive in nature, able to care for most of the medical and surgical, as well as the rehabilitative, needs of the residents/patients. What distinguishes them most is that they adhere to a rehabilitation, rather than a medical, model of treatment. When surgery is performed, for example, it is corrective in nature and medical treatment is aimed at controlling seizures, reducing pain and inflammation of body joints, and so on. When acute medical treatment is necessary, such as an emergency appendectomy, a disabled person might be operated upon within the rehabilitation setting but would more often be transferred to a general medical hospital for the surgery.

If Eleanor's corrective surgery had been performed within a comprehensive medical rehabilitation setting, she would have gone immediately from the postoperative stage into the active rehabilitation process. As a result, she most likely would have been discharged at a higher level of independent functioning and, with appropriate home services, within a shorter period of time.

From a disabled person's point of view, the differences between the various medical rehabilitation settings are significant. For example, the staff in a comprehensive setting are acutely aware that severely disabled people require certain services that nondisabled people in general medical settings may not. Staff within a general medical setting are often poorly informed about the special needs of the severely disabled, and so may discount a disabled patient's request for certain services. In addition, general medical hospitals are usually too understaffed to render the amount and the quality of nursing care some severely disabled people require. An SCI patient's claim that he must be turned in bed frequently, day and night, or otherwise he might develop decubitus ulcers may, therefore, be ignored. This is one reason why severely disabled patients who are transferred to medical rehabilitation facilities from general medical hospitals often arrive in serious condition.

In Tennessee, a 16-year-old girl who broke her neck in an auto accident was sent to a small rural hospital for six weeks before being transferred to a rehabilitation annex in Memphis. By the time she arrived at the annex, she had developed 16 decubitus ulcers, 4 of which were serious enough to require skin grafts. Because of similar medical disasters, former residents/patients of medical rehabilitation facilities, when they require acute medical care, very often request that they be treated within, or be transferred back as quickly as possible to, the facility, where they know they can depend on appropriate care.

Another advantage of comprehensive medical rehabilitation settings is that they facilitate the transfer of self-care skills learned in therapy sessions to the activities that disabled residents/patients engage in outside of therapy. It is difficult for people who are severely disabled and who spend a limited number of hours each day learning self-care and homemaking skills to feel confident enough to rely on those skills once they leave their therapy sessions. And their self-confidence is not increased if, outside of therapy, staff members assist them in performing activities they are struggling to learn to perform independently. In comprehensive medical rehabilitation settings, ADL skills are more likely to be retained and improved because residents/patients are expected to practice what they learn in therapy when they get back to their living quarters. In more limited medical rehabilitation settings, general medical treatment policies tend to prevail, and these policies may work against the requisite transfer of ADL skills.

For example, John W., an SCI quadriplegic in a Midwest Veterans Hospital, had received permission from the chief of staff to try using a new type of suppository inserter. If John could have mastered the use of the inserter, he would have been independent in his bowel management. The first time John tried using the inserter, however, he was stopped before he could succeed. The nurse who was assigned to help him with his bowel care that day took the inserter away from John and completed the procedure herself, saying she didn't have any time to waste waiting for him. In her daily report, she wrote that John was unable to successfully use the inserter, a conclusion she arrived at after five minutes of impatient observation. Fortunately, in John's case his determination to become independent resulted in his learning to use the inserter with his mother's help, but only after he was discharged.

In medical rehabilitation facilities where the rehabilitation model of treatment prevails, the needs of disabled people are given higher priority than the needs of staff members. Here severely disabled people, like John, receive the encouragement they need to persist in their attempts to learn self-care skills, whether or not the staff is convinced they can succeed. While factors of safety and patient morale may mean a halt in the individual's efforts, factors of staff time and convenience do not.

## STAGES OF MEDICAL REHABILITATION

Many variations occur within the medical rehabilitation process from one setting to another and from one disability type to another. The rehabilitation process may vary depending on (1) the type of disability concerned, (2) whether the disability is congenital or acquired, (3) whether the disability is stable or progressive, and (4) whether the disability is moderate or severe. Other variations result from limitations on available resources and, perhaps most importantly, from differences in the prevailing treatment philosophies in different settings. While most medical rehabilitation professionals support the global goals of medical rehabilitation in principle, the financial exigencies facing the entire field of rehabilitation often force those who are in a position to dictate service policies to divert limited staff and facility resources from role restoration to physical restoration efforts. Despite these variations it is convenient for discussion purposes to divide the overall medical rehabilitation process into four distinct stages.

### STAGE ONE: ACUTE MEDICAL CARE

During the initial stage of the medical rehabilitation process, the emphasis is on treating the precipitating cause of the disabling condition. Most often this stage takes place somewhere other than in a medical rehabilitation setting. When Ernie broke his neck, he was rushed to a general medical hospital where he remained until his condition stabilized and he could be transferred safely to a regional medical rehabilitation center. Like many, the general medical hospital in which Ernie found himself lacked staff with specialized training or experience in treating people with spinal cord injuries. One side-effect of their inadequate training seemed inconsequential at the time when Ernie's life was in jeopardy, but later proved to have long-lasting, serious consequences for his eventual psychological adjustment.

Their lack of experience resulted in the staff believing—and passing the belief on to Ernie's parents—that, if Ernie lived, he would lead a restricted, unfulfilling existence and would never be free of the need for constant attendant care. While subsequent rehabilitation efforts resulted in Ernie becoming self-sufficient in his self-care, his parents were unable to free themselves of the conviction that they were responsible for Ernie's support and daily living needs. Trapped by their conviction and Ernie's expectations, they continued to absolve him of all responsibility for managing his own life. Only after Ernie decided to marry and establish a home of his own did the cycle of dependency–overprotectiveness, leading to greater dependency, begin to be broken. Even his proven self-sufficiency within a medical rehabilitation setting had failed to alter either his own or his parents' beliefs and expectations.

Persons who work in general medical settings tend to be overwhelmed by what they perceive to be the inevitable consequences of a permanent injury to the spinal cord. They may have had no experience with the treatment possibilities for people with spinal cord injury to counteract their own feelings of helplessness and hopelessness (DeLoach and Greer, 1981; Mitchell, 1976). Within a specialized medical setting, on the other hand, along with acute medical treatment, procedures that simplify the subsequent rehabilitation process are initiated. In the case of spinal cord injury, for example, in addition to administering antibiotics and stabilizing the spinal column, medical rehabilitation personnel knowledgeable about the effects of spinal cord injury would prescribe high-calorie diets containing a mimimum of 150 grams of protein daily and administer anabolic hormones to prevent unnecessary tissue breakdown and to help stabilize basic body functions (Rusk, 1977).

When the acute stage takes place within a nonspecialized medical setting, normal complications may be exacerbated, due to an overriding concern with life-saving techniques and procedures. With disabilities as disparate as spinal cord injury and myocardial infarction (heart attack), attention paid at the outset to basic psychosocial aspects of the disabling condition can enhance the overall rehabilitation process, by laying the foundation for a person's eventual reentry into community life while that person is still acutely ill.

According to Wright (1960), Cobb (1973), and DeLoach and Greer (1981), the two psychological reactions most detrimental to desired rehabilitation outcomes are unrealistic hope and unrealistic fear. While the role that either reaction plays varies with the nature of the disabling condition, in order to forestall the detrimental effects of either reaction on an individual's eventual physical, psychological and social adjustment, medical and paramedical professionals who come in contact with the individual need to be acquainted from the first with the entire rehabilitation process.

For example, no medical miracles occur after the integrity of a spinal cord has been completely destroyed at the point of a spinal cord injury. If the spinal cord has not been destroyed completely, however, and certain neural pathways are still intact, the pattern and permanence of body paralysis and sensory loss are difficult to predict accurately. In some cases physical function may return, either partially or completely.

Unfortunately, sometimes medical professionals who do not specialize in spinal cord injury forget what they once learned about ·`e complex nature of paralysis. Paralysis is not synonymous with e inability to move; paralysis is the inability to move voluntarily. The involuntary movement of paralyzed skeletal muscles following complete cord injuries may confuse disabled people and their families, unless they are prepared by medical professionals for the normal sequence of events that follow such injuries.

In affected portions of the body, spinal cord isjury results in spastic paralysis, where sensory nerve impulses entering the cord from the periphery of the body still synapse (make contact) with the motor neurons that extend from the cord back out to where they cause a reaction in muscle fibers or some other microscopic body parts. This reflex arc, consisting of sensory and motor nerve cells, is intact in the portion of the cord below the point of injury and results in movement, usually excessive movement called spasms. But because motor-sensory pathways from the cord to the brain are blocked at the damaged area of the cord, movement below the damaged area can neither be initiated nor be stopped by the higher brain centers that normally control skeletal muscle movement.

Immediately after the spinal cord is injured, the portion of the cord at and below the point of injury goes into shock and is, therefore, incapable of responding to any stimuli, so no movement, voluntary or involuntary, can occur in paralyzed body parts. After this period of spinal shock passes, however, reflex activity resumes below the point of injury, and paralyzed limbs apparently regain their ability to move. This resumption of involuntary movement—that is, spastic paralysis—usually occurs during the acute stage of medical treatment. If the disabled person is in a general medical hospital and no rehabilitation specialists are available, patient and family may misinterpret this return of movement as an indication that recovery is occurring, and they may not have their misinterpretation corrected.

The impact of spastic paralysis, like the absence of pain that often follows a heart attack, is compounded by the fact that people's first psychological defense following the onset of a disability is denial: denial, first, that the disabling incident occurred and, second, that the disabling effects will be permanent. Unrealistic hope—that is, denial—can jeopardize the success of subsequent medical rehabilitation or ILR efforts, because the patients believe their eventual recovery makes any rehabilitation service unnecessary (Cobb, 1973).

Irrational fear may be as detrimental to the rehabilitation of cardiac patients as false hope is to the spinal cord injured. A heart attack is frightening in itself, especially since the person having it is aware that he or she could die. Added to this initial fear reaction is the possibility that persons who have experienced severe heart attacks will develop what has become known as ICU psychosis—a psychological aberration stemming from the medications and sensory overloads common to intensive care units. The result of these psychological factors is that, following a myocardial infarction, many people avoid participating in any activities that they fear could provoke another, possibly fatal, attack.

These adverse psychological factors can be controlled more effectively in settings where medical rehabilitation professionals are involved in the acute stage of medical treatment than in situations where unrealistic hopes and fears prevail. Although the main concern in the acute stage is the survival of the newly disabled person, the overall rehabilitation process will be aided if, as soon as the patient's condition has stabilized, the various professionals who will be providing rehabilitation services to the patient make introductory visits. Early contact, especially with a vocational rehabilitation counselor, will help patients realize that their lives are not over and that they may return to gainful employment.

## STAGE TWO: PHYSICAL RESTORATION

After a newly disabled person's vital signs have stabilized, concern is focused on optimum physiological recovery and on determining the person's medical and rehabilitation potential. In this second stage of the medical rehabilitation process, rehabilitation therapists assume a central role in the treatment program, along with physicians who specialize in the various affected body systems. Together, physicians and therapists begin to assess the extent and the permanency of neural or cardiac damage (to use the examples developed above), and to design a rehabilitation program that will maintain or enhance the remaining physical function to the greatest degree possible. Radiologic studies of the spinal column, along with muscle and range-of-motion tests, help determine whether a spinal cord injury is complete or incomplete and the pattern of neural damage. Electrocardiograms, in conjunction with tests of heart tolerance, help establish safe levels of physical activity consistent with a damaged heart.

Hopefully, even in settings with limited medical rehabilitation services, patients' muscles will have been kept conditioned and their joints flexible. While patients are acutely ill, therapeutic procedures can be carried out that exercise their arms, legs, hands, and feet while they remain passive. During this second stage, however, patients become active participants in their therapeutic regimens. For people like Ernie, this means that they actively carry out exercises designed to increase the strength of those muscles that remain under voluntary control and learn to carry out the proper positioning procedures to prevent tightening of joints or the development of decubitus ulcers in paralyzed body parts. For someone who has sustained damage of the heart muscle, this stage entails closely supervised, daily increments in physical activity until the upper margins of safe energy expenditure have been reached.

Although all the various medical rehabilitation professionals are more actively involved in a treatment program in stage two than in stage one, it is not until stage three that the professionals who specialize in psychosocial aspects of rehabilitation begin to assume a central role. In medical rehabilitation programs with minimal staffs, stage two frequently marks the conclusion of effective medical rehabilitation efforts, because services that might allow severely disabled people to reach their optimum levels of independent functioning are not available.

## STAGE THREE: INTENSIVE MEDICAL REHABILITATION

Stage three is the stage where disabled people are given the training and equipment they need to function as effectively as they can in a world designed primarily for people who are not disabled. In stage three, medical rehabilitation professionals work as a team, pooling their expertise in an all-out effort to help patients attain their rehabilitation goals. This use of an onsite team is the hallmark of medical rehabilitation. It is impossible to overstate the importance of patient and staff availability to the success of the medical rehabilitation process, for unlike other rehabilitation professionals, those who work with inpatients in a medical rehabilitation setting do not have to compete with external demands on their patients' time and energy. In the temporary world of a rehabilitation facility, the goal of patients is to be rehabilitated, and the main task of the rehabilitation team is assisting patients to attain that goal. When patients live outside a facility setting, on any single day they may see their primary obligation as any one of innumerable obligations unrelated to their primary rehabilitation goals. To a large degree, then, control of patients' environments is an important step in assisting them to establish control over their own lives.

While the team approach is characteristic of all categories of rehabilitation services, coordination of rehabilitation efforts among people who work in scattered sites differs fundamentally from the onsite teamwork that typifies the medical rehabilitation process. First, in medical rehabilitation team members tend to work within the same facility, which increases their ability to communicate and, consequently, their professional effectiveness. Second, team members are in daily contact with the one indispensable member of the team, the patient himself.

Because optimum rehabilitation, whether medical or not, is designed to restore people to their highest level of functioning in every aspect of their lives, a wide variety of skills and expertise is required among those who work with disabled people in a rehabilitative context. Just what professionals are represented in a particular rehabilitation effort, however, depends primarily on the nature of the disabling condition. While some authorities claim that a viable team can consist of a physician, a nurse, a rehabilitation therapist, and a social worker, most medical rehabilitation experts believe such a limited team would result in severely disabled people functioning far beneath their potential (Rusk, 1977). Unfortunately, inadequate staffs exist in many settings, with the result that many severely physically disabled people conclude their medical rehabilitation at a lower level of independent functioning than their condition warrants (Bowe, 1978; DeLoach and Greer, 1981).

Depending on the type of disability involved, the following rehabilitation professions could be represented on a medical rehabilitation team (Rusk, 1977).

1. A physiatrist who specializes in physical medicine and rehabilitation.

2. Any other medical specialist whose speciality is important in the rehabilitation of disabled people. For example, in the case of spinal cord injury, Rusk (1977) recommends that a neurosurgeon, a urologist, an orthopedic surgeon, an internist, a neurologist and a psychiatrist be included on the team. In the case of cardiac disabilities, he recommends a cardiologist and, in certain cases, a cardiac surgeon.

3. A rehabilitation nurse who ensures that the skills learned in therapy are practiced outside of therapy and that other types of therapeutic regimens are also carried out within the daily hospital routine.

4. A physical therapist who is trained in the use of a wide range of treatment modalities, such as heat, cold, and ultrasound, and who trains patients in the use of mobility aids and techniques.

5. An occupational therapist who specializes in techniques designed to improve fine motor coordination and who teaches patients techniques and provides adaptive aids that allow them to perform their ADL.

6. A social worker who assists patients and their families to use community resources to ameliorate the financial, housing, and social problems created by the existence of a disabling condition.

7. A psychologist who assists patients with their psychological adjustment.

8. A rehabilitation counselor who provides career planning, training, and placement services.

9. A recreation therapist who helps patients to reestablish their community living skills and to develop self-satisfying leisure-time activities.

10. A number of other professionals, such as audiologists, speech therapists, orthotists (brace makers), and prosthetists (artificial limb makers), whose services may be needed to formulate programs and to treat people with certain disabling conditions. For instance, in cardiac rehabilitation a medical technologist administers electrocardiograms and tests of heart tolerance.

Although certain members of the team begin working with patients during the acute stage, it is during the intensive stage that the team approach dominates the rehabilitation process. In concert with patients, team members formulate rehabilitation goals and strive to make those goals a reality. At this stage in the process, the emphasis begins to shift from primarily physical restoration efforts to efforts aimed at role restoration—efforts, that is, that are intended to help patients cope with the demands of living outside a sheltered setting. During this stage, team energies are directed toward helping disabled people find suitable accommodations, providing them with training in ADL, and referring them to appropriate community and government agencies to ensure continuity of services after the conclusion of the active medical rehabilitation process.

For some disabled people, the goal of rehabilitation may be placement in a suitable nursing home. For others, the goal may be employment and physical self-sufficiency. But however effective a medical rehabilitation effort may be, the team will find it impossible to bring severely disabled people to their optimum levels of functioning within the brief time that they are involved in the onsite rehabilitation process. Even for newly disabled SCI patients, the period of time spent as an inpatient receiving medical rehabilitation rarely exceeds 120 days. Within this period, SCI patients may learn basic skills, but they may require years of practice before they can develop those skills to the maximum. Moreover, disabled people return to different communities, each of which will offer a unique set of challenges for which the medical rehabilitation process is unable to prepare them. In most instances, for example, the exact skills a person requires to cope in a particular living situation will not become apparent until he or she has returned home and lived there for some time.

Because medical rehabilitation is an expensive process, both in terms of the time expended by a variety of rehabilitation professionals and in terms of the sophisticated equipment and facilities used to provide needed services, medical rehabilitation services must be offered in an intensive, time-limited program that can only begin to provide the groundwork required for severely disabled people to build full, productive lives. Moreover, medical rehabilitation suffers from a perpetual lack of adequate funding and a shortage of qualified, experienced personnel, and so cannot provide, on an inpatient basis, the duration of services that severely disabled people require.

## STAGE FOUR: FOLLOW-UP SERVICES

In the fourth stage of the medical rehabilitation process, the team maintains contact with recently discharged people, in order to monitor their progress and to provide whatever additional services are needed. In most cases this fourth stage exists only in theory, for few medical rehabilitation programs have the resources to offer effective follow-up services. Instead of periodically visiting former patients in their home settings, a medical rehabilitation team may be able to visit patients' homes only once prior to their discharge, in order to detect and remedy any problems in the home environment. Simply asking newly disabled people if they anticipate any difficulty entering their homes, for example, does not preclude the need for home visits by experienced professionals. The majority of people will not remember the existence of architectural barriers that were of no consequence to them before they became disabled. This lack of follow-up service often results in disabled people with recently acquired self-care and community reentry skills being unable to exercise those skills after their discharge from medical rehabilitation programs.

Even under optimal circumstances, however, the medical rehabilitation process is not intended to meet the long-term IL needs of severely disabled people. For this reason community-based IL programs have evolved to complement medical rehabilitation programs and to ensure that progress toward independent lifestyles achieved during the medical rehabilitation process is not lost once that process ends.

## MEDICALLY BASED DETERRENTS TO INDEPENDENT LIVING

The very nature of the medical rehabilitation model means that it produces certain deterrents that work against severely disabled people establishing optimally independent lifestyles. First, because it is based on the medical model of treatment, medical rehabilitation often inhibits the development of behaviors that are essential to severely disabled people's ability to live independently. Second, because most medical rehabilitation programs are unable to provide adequate follow-up services, people who are vulnerable to sudden changes in the state of their health or living conditions are denied services that might lessen the risks associated with an independent lifestyle, which leads them to avoid independence-enhancing behaviors.

AUTHORITARIAN NATURE OF THE MEDICAL MODEL

Because medical rehabilitation is a speciality within the field of medicine, medical rehabilitation professionals and paraprofessionals are imbued with the authoritarian philosophy of treatment that typifies medical training in general. In part, the authoritarianism inherent in the philosophy of medical treatment is due to the fact that most physicians believe, and medical students are taught, that the two essential ingredients in a successful physician-patient relationship are the physician's authority over the patient and the patient's acceptance of that authority (Pratt, Seligman, and Reader, 1958; Stein, 1978). In part, this authoritarianism is due to the fact that people in medically related professions have had years of training and experience that their patients do not, and, therefore, they find it easy to justify the authoritarian-physician–submissive-patient paradigm of medical treatment. In actual fact, however, McKinley (1975) has demonstrated that medical professionals underestimate the medical knowledge of even those patients with little formal education.

Although the accepted authority of a physician may be efficacious in the treatment of people with acute illness, it can be detrimental (see Chapter 6) in the treatment of people who have successfully coped with the medical ramifications of a disabling condition for a long period of time. When one is acutely ill, treatment decisions must often be arrived at quickly and any question as to appropriateness of treatment is often best resolved through consultation with other medical experts. But the situation is altered when medical decisions relate to the treatment of a disabling condition with which a patient has had years of personal experience (DeLoach and Greer, 1981; Richardson, 1972).

While it is obvious that disabled people are subject to the entire range of acute disorders that afflict the nondisabled, it should also be obvious that, unless they are to spend the rest of their lives in custodial care, disabled people must assume some responsibility for their medical management in areas related to their disabling conditions. Those who cannot or will not assume such responsibility cannot thrive living within the community, because to do so they must practice proper medical self-management and monitor their physiological functioning periodically to detect and forestall any preventable medical problems.

Unfortunately, medical rehabilitation policies tend to encourage passive behaviors and discourage assertive behaviors in medically related areas. But if the medical rehabilitation process is to enhance the living potentials of those whom it serves, it must first incorporate basic medical information and self-management techniques into its treatment program and then prepare patients for their encounters in the future with physicians who may be unaware of the physiological complications common to many disabling conditions (Berman, 1978). Only by replacing the medical model of treatment with a rehabilitative model (see Chapter 6) can the rehabilitation process develop the self-assertive behaviors that have proven to be highly correlated with satisfactory results in rehabilitation (Kerr, 1970; Ramsey, 1978; Richardson, 1972; Vineberg and Willems, 1971; Weinberg and Williams, 1978).

# 6

# Community-Based Medical Services and Independent Living

If disabled people of any age are to maintain optimum levels of independent functioning outside medical or custodial environments, they must not only attain some degree of physiological stability, but also assume some degree of responsibility for their continuing health care. In order to lessen the difficulties of obtaining appropriate medical care after they are no longer engaged in the active medical rehabilitation process, they first must have confidence that they are capable of medical self-management and then must convince others of their expertise in areas directly related to their disabling conditions.

Unfortunately, the social myth—stemming from societal definitions of health and illness in our society (Parsons, 1958, chap. 3)—that people who are disabled are incapable of managing their own lives imposes as severe a handicap on disabled people as do their physical limitations (Bowe, 1978; DeLoach and Greer, 1981; Hale, 1979). The tendency to discount the ability of people who are disabled to make valid decisions in matters directly concerning them is not limited to the general public but is preva-

**113**

lent in the general medical community (Kerr, 1972; Richardson, 1972).

Physicians with no special training or experience in rehabilitation medicine often view all those requiring health care as medically unsophisticated (McKinley, 1975). Such physicians may make no distinction between people who require treatment for acute illnesses and those who have lived and dealt with the physical ramifications of a disabling condition for a considerable period of time and who, therefore, may know more about their routine treatment needs than many general medical practitioners. Nevertheless, physically disabled people must rely on the general medical community for the medications, physical examinations, and specialized health care they require but, too often, do not obtain.

This chapter will

1. discuss the treatment needs of disabled or chronically ill people who must obtain their medical care within the general medical community,

2. discuss the need for all medical and paramedical personnel to have some training in rehabilitation medicine,

3. suggest ways in which disabled and chronically ill people can reduce their dependency on general medical practitioners,

4. recommend methods of improving the quality of the care that disabled and chronically ill people receive in community medical settings.

The medical needs of severely physically disabled people who live within their communities differ from the needs of other community members in several ways. First, disabled people tend to require more ongoing medical care than do nondisabled people. Second, disabled people, on the average, spend a larger percentage of their family income on disability-related medical expenses. Third, disabled people need to be treated by health professionals who have some experience with the complications common to specific disabling conditions. Fourth, disabled people find it difficult to obtain the quality of medical services they require.

## COST AND EXTENT OF REQUIRED MEDICAL CARE

Most severely disabled people accumulate yearly medical bills that would overwhelm people whose medical expenses are limited to the cost of periodic medical and dental examinations. A large percentage of many disabled people's total expenditure on disability-related medical expenses is for prescribed medications they take on a continuous basis. For example, people who sustain brain damage in auto accidents or from cerebral vascular accidents (CVA)—that is, strokes—often develop, along with possible sensory, motor, or judgmental deficits, a seizure disorder. They, like the 30 percent or more of those with cerebral palsy who also experience seizures or who are seizure-prone, may require medications to control their seizures for as long as they live. People with other neurological disabilities, such as multiple sclerosis or spinal cord injury, tend to be susceptible to chronic urinary infections. Therefore, such people should have urinary function tests at least once a year to prevent potentially irreversible damage to their kidneys and may need to remain on some lifelong regimen of maintenance drugs to prevent chronic infections from getting out of control. In short, for most people with permanent disabilities, medications, whether to control or prevent seizure activity, reduce muscle spasticity, reduce pain and swelling in joints, or combat and control infections, tend to be a fixed expense in their family budgets.

Other atypical medical expenses of the disabled arise from their more frequent need for medical care. While the health of many disabled people rivals that of their nondisabled contemporaries, the percentage requiring medical treatment for acute or chronic conditions is higher than in the general population (Goldenson et al., 1978).

This is especially true for those with spinal cord injury. According to Young and Northup (1980, p. 21), "grievous, permanent disturbances of the neuro-muscular, neuro-sensory, cardiopulmonary, gastro-intestinal, genito-urinary, endocrine and other systems, predispose the spinal cord injured person to subsequent deterioration—medically, psychologically and socially." Young and Northup base this claim on the results of their studies of representative samples of people with spinal cord injuries. When reviewing how often their subjects were hospitalized in the second and third years following the onset of their injuries, Young and Northup discovered that, while there was a great deal of variation among individuals, a substantial percentage were hospitalized each year.

For example, in the second year following their injury, paraplegics and quadriplegics in the sample were hospitalized for periods ranging from 0 to 250 days. In the third year following their injury, they were hospitalized for 0 to 210 days. According to Young and Northup, however, an "amazingly large group . . .

required no hospitalization in Years Two and Three." Nevertheless, despite the trend toward less hospitalization the longer the subjects had been disabled, a high percentage required intensive medical treatment sometime during both their second and third years.

What differentiates spinal cord injured people who require hospitalization from those who do not? In the Young and Northup studies, the number of days of hospitalization required correlated most highly with how well the disabled person coped with the ramifications—physical, psychological and social—of his or her disabilities. According to Young and Northup, there is a significant relationship between people's general coping skills and their state of health, while there is little or no relationship between type or severity of disability and health. Young and Northup claim that those who do not fare well medically usually have problems dealing with their disabilities in their daily lives, since "the extent to which a disabled person achieves an enjoyable, meaningful lifestyle will logically vary directly with the maintenance of good health. Most certainly the medical and social costs associated with an individual's disability are markedly influenced by the state of health of that person" (p. 25).

In addition to the expenses they incur obtaining medications and intermittent intensive medical treatment, severely disabled people also spend extraordinary amounts of money in other disability-related areas, such as adaptive equipment and environmental modifications. Young and Northup (1979) compiled the following data concerning the cost of (1) physicians' care; (2) prescribed medications; (3) adaptive equipment; and (4) needed environmental modifications for (a) the year in which a disability occurred and (b) the second and third years following a disabling incident.

In the year during which they became disabled, people with spinal cord injuries on the average, incurred these expenses for medical services: $3,640 for physicians' fees; $1,527 for medication and medical supplies; $2,194 for adaptive equipment; and $1,786 for environmental modifications. By the end of the first year, the average total expenditure for *only* these four categories of disability-related medical expenses was $9,147, of which $5,188 was incurred during the time the subjects were inpatients undergoing medical rehabilitation. These four categories alone, which do not include the cost of hospital rooms, physical and occupational therapy, and so on, accounted for nearly one-fourth the overall average first year medical costs of $38,117.

The fact that initial medical costs for newly disabled people are extremely high is not surprising. What is pertinent to the relationship between IL services and community-based medical services is the high cost of medical care for severely disabled people after they have concluded their active medical rehabilitation. For an indication of how much of their available income people who are not covered by a third party payer must devote to their health care needs, Young and Northup investigated the medical expenses of their subjects in the second and third years after they became disabled. In the second year, spinal cord injured patients, on the average, paid $628 for physicians' fees; $669 for medication and supplies; $550 for adaptive equipment; and $1,030 for environmental modifications. In the third year, they paid, on the average, $559 for physicians' fees; $615 for medication and supplies; $346 for adaptive equipment; and $586 for environmental modifications.

Although, according to the above studies, the need for medical care and the cost of certain medical services decreases over time, some disability-related medical expenses increase because of the rising cost of health care in general. Take, for example, the cost of specific types of commonly required adaptive equipment and the expenses incurred in maintaining that equipment. In the late 1970s, a standard, 24-volt Everest and Jennings power wheelchair could be purchased for approximately $2,000. By 1981, the same type of power wheelchair, with a few minor improvements, cost approximately $3,000.

Another disability-related medical expense often overlooked in estimates of average costs involves the repair and maintenance of adaptive equipment. According to statistics compiled by the Berkeley CIL (*Wheelchair II Conference Proceedings*, 1979), the average yearly repair cost for a power wheelchair, not counting labor, was $600 in 1979, and in 1981 the cost of labor alone was approximately $20 an hour. Because of the expense of repairing and maintaining sophisticated adaptive equipment, in addition to the difficulty of finding someone who can repair it, many disabled people are unable to utilize the technological aids designed to help them live more independently. While some private and public organizations and agencies will purchase a variety of adaptive aids for severely disabled people, most will not underwrite repair and maintenance costs. For this reason, many environmental control systems, computerized reading machines, teletypewriters, or customized wheelchairs are not used by the people for whom they were intended, because these people cannot afford the cost of operating them (Anderson, 1977; Bruck, 1978).

## DIFFICULTY IN OBTAINING
## APPROPRIATE MEDICAL SERVICES

While few disabled people realize it at the time, the period during which they are actively engaged in the medical rehabilitation process is often the halcyon period of their newly established relationship with the medical community. Although the medical model of treatment, which predominates in some medical rehabilitation facilities, may be detrimental to the psychosocial adjustment of newly disabled people, the presence of well-trained, experienced medical rehabilitation professionals is beneficial to their overall physical wellbeing (Margolin, 1971).

During the time newly disabled people are being treated in medical rehabilitation facilities, they are shielded from medical practices that might result in secondary disabilities or exacerbate the complications of primary disabling conditions. For example, rehabilitation nurses guard against the development of decubitus ulcers by making certain that patients do not remain in one position for too long. In addition, along with other members of the medical rehabilitation team, they train patients in proper methods of medical self-management, such as the proper procedures for changing and irrigating catheters.

Once they have completed their active medical rehabilitation and have been discharged from the rehabilitation facility, however, severely disabled people become dependent for their intensive medical treatment on members of the general medical community. It is only after being discharged that most discover that not all medical personnel are as cognizant of their unique treatment requirements as were the medical personnel in the medical rehabilitation facility. When they begin to look for a physician and medical facilities in their communities, they often discover that not all physicians are willing to accept disabled people as patients and that not all medical facilities are accessible. Moreover, in many instances they can no longer avail themselves of the services of a medical rehabilitation facility, even as outpatients.

Although the fourth stage of the medical rehabilitation process was designed to provide follow-up services to former patients, staff and financial constraints often result in follow-up services being eliminated or being too attenuated to effectively meet the medical needs of people who have been discharged and who have returned to their home communities. The reason is that most comprehensive medical rehabilitation facilities attempt to maintain a 20 to 40 bed capacity for each major disability type served, which cost-effectiveness studies indicate is the optimum number (Young and Northup, 1979). Therefore, in order to operate at maximum efficiency, most facilities are forced to draw patients from a wide geographical area to keep the optimum number of beds filled. As a result, many disabled people, after they complete the active phase of their medical rehabilitation, return to towns and rural areas located far from the facility. In such cases, distance makes it difficult for the medical rehabilitation team to effectively monitor and evaluate their progress.

Once in the general community, disabled people discover that few physicians have had adequate experience with patients with different types and degrees of disability. Medicine is so vast and complex a discipline that the old medical school joke—"A medical specialist is someone who knows practically everything about practically nothing, while a general practitioner is someone who knows practically nothing about practically everything"—is especially appropriate to the treatment of the disabled. What disabled people require is a personal physician who knows practically everything about the disability in question but who also knows practically everything about anything that can become or create a secondary disabling condition.

Unfortunately, even the most conservative estimate of 26 million disabled in the United States, if broken down into disability types, presents an impossible challenge to even the most dedicated medical practitioner. For example, approximately 10 million people in the United States are significantly disabled from a disorder affecting the musculoskeletal system alone (Hylbert and Hylbert, 1979), but there are over one thousand different disorders that affect the musculoskeletal system. More than 160 different arthritic conditions have been identified, each with varied etiologies (causes) and physiological effects. What physician in general practice, especially in a small community with limited access to colleagues who specialize in rheumatology, can even be expected to competently treat all those who consult him or her about their "arthritis"? Add to this the fact that the majority of physicians in practice today completed their medical training over ten years ago, and it is not surprising that physicians sometimes make inappropriate treatment decisions (Berman, 1978).

Among the most serious medical hazards facing disabled people who seek medical treatment in the general community are the potentially dangerous interactions of newly prescribed medications with medications that were previously prescribed to treat certain disabling conditions. For example, people with chronic conditions, such as epilepsy, have had medications prescribed that interact with the medications taken to control symptoms of the primary disabling condition, such as seizures, causing the seizures to recur. Moreover, many medications prescribed to ameliorate the effects of a disabling condition may be themselves potentially life-threatening.

Even over-the-counter drugs, such as aspirin, can produce serious side-effects in people who are unusually sensitive to them, and many prescribed drugs are, to some degree, toxic for everyone. Complicating an already complicated issue is the fact that people tend to build up a tolerance to medication they have taken for a long period, so that a drug that produced the desired effect when it was first prescribed may gradually lose its effectiveness or may accumulate in the body, eventually destroying vital body tissues. Adverse reactions to commonly prescribed drugs can range from the stultifying effects of drugs used in seizure control to the addictive effects of drugs used to control spasticity of skeletal muscles.

It is not unusual for the effects of inappropriate or inadequately monitored treatment efforts to be as incapacitating as the original disabling condition. Yet even inappropriate or inadequately monitored medical treatment may not be available to many disabled people in our society. The extent of the health care problem facing disabled people was reflected in the agenda of the 1977 White House Conference on Handicapped Individuals, a large segment of which was devoted to health and health care concerns. According to the summary of the proceedings, "Conference participants expressed concern about the lack of *affordable,* locally *available,* diagnostic, treatment and referral services in nonrestrictive, culturally oriented and *accessible* service facilities" (*White House Conference on Handicapped Individuals,* 1978, p. 219).

These concerns voiced on the national level repeated the concerns previously expressed by leaders in the field of medical rehabilitation. These physicians believe medical rehabilitation "can and should be carried out by the general practitioner or specialist responsible for the patient's primary medical care" (Swinyard et al., 1977, p. 78), for "without incorporating basic medical rehabilitation procedures into regular medical approaches to the treatment of the disabled and elderly, further but unnecessary deterioration and increased disability among the great majority of our sick and injured can be expected." Furthermore, according to Swinyard et al., the reason an effort should be made to incorporate medical rehabilitation procedures into general medical practice is that most of the medical services available to disabled people are rendered in physicians' offices or in general medical hospitals instead of in specialized medical rehabilitation settings.

But even if basic rehabilitation procedures were incorporated into general medical services, the health care needs of severely disabled people still might not be met. Adequate health care for such people depends on a network of community support services, in which the lack of one can disrupt the effectiveness of all other services within the network. Among the support services most vital to the health care needs of disabled people are accessible public transportation, accessible health care facilities, appropriate health maintenance organizations, and adequate income maintenance programs.

The lack of accessible public transportation, which will be discussed in depth in Chapter 8, continues to be a major obstacle to adequate health care for many disabled individuals. In 1977 an estimated 17.5 million people had disabilities severe enough to prevent them from using unmodified public transportation (Mace, 1977). In the 1980s the transportation problem was compounded by the bankruptcy of many large urban mass-transit systems. Lack of accessible public transportation results in many people being unable to obtain the medical services they require.

People who are unable to use unmodified public transportation services are also usually unable to utilize medical services in facilities that are not barrier-free. Although progress was made in barrier removal during the last half of the 1970s, in part due to Section 504 of the 1973 Rehabilitation Act, the Reagan administration's drive to reduce federal regulations and funding virtually eliminated federally based incentives for barrier removal.

Often, however, even in facilities that had attempted to abide by government regulations, lack of understanding of what accessibility entails or of adherence to accessibility codes resulted in barrier-removal projects that reduced but did not eliminate existing barriers. For example, in Chicago the front entrance to the Art Institute had a ramp that ended in a series of steps, making the entrance still inaccessible to wheelchairs. In Boston a curb-cut leading from a parking lot to an office building has a light standard in the middle of it that prevents anyone with a mobility impairment from passing. In Memphis, the Baptist Memorial Hospital has two public restrooms that were modified for people in wheelchairs but that are unusable by anyone using a wheelchair. One small restroom has a wide door that opens inward, so that once a person in a wheelchair enters, he cannot close the door past the wheelchair. The other restroom has a privacy baffle outside the restroom entrance that is too close to the entrance to allow a wheelchair to pass.

## CONSEQUENCES OF UNMET HEALTH CARE NEEDS

The consequences for disabled people of insufficient medical services include deterioration of their overall state of health, development of additional disabling conditions and, in some instances, a shortened life. When needed prescription changes do not occur, once-sensitive organisms may become immune to medications that have been taken for long periods, and infections that were once easily controlled may become virulent, or adverse drug reactions may go undetected until irreversible tissue changes occur in the liver, kidneys, or cardiovascular system.

Although in some instances, disabled people may fail to follow prescribed medical regimens or may not take advantage of the medical services that are available, in most cases needed medical services are not available, with the result that "children are still found in their homes undiagnosed and untreated, amputees still walk the street without prostheses, discharged patients still sit in their homes unable to get out, lacking transportation, funds, jobs and accessible housing" (Swinyard et al., 1977, p. 87). Lack of comprehensive, long-term medical services also results in many clients of IL programs arriving at their initial interviews suffering from the effects of inadequate medical care.

When Joel H., a 27-year-old who had sustained a cervical injury in a waterskiing accident, was discharged from a medical rehabilitation center, he was independent in his self-care and was judged to be well-adjusted psychologically and socially. Joel returned home to a small rural community that had one physician, a general medical practitioner, who treated Joel's minor medical problems to the best of his ability but who had to refer Joel to a medical center 60 miles away for more intensive medical treatment.

At the time Joel, who had moved to be closer to the medical center, applied for IL services he had had both legs amputated, as a result of recurring decubitus ulcers, and had permanent loss of kidney function, due to repeated urinary infections. Perhaps as a result of his additional disabilities, Joel had lost nearly all of his self-care skills, but retained the ability to wipe his face, put on his hat and wheel his chair for short distances on a smooth, level surface. With the services he received through the IL program, Joel eventually regained his self-care skills, but IL services could do nothing to restore his legs or repair the damage done to his kidneys.

Would Joel have had fewer physical disabilities, and would he have continued to function more independently than he did when he applied for IL services, if the medical care he had received after he left the medical rehabilitation center had been designed to prevent the potential complications of a spinal cord injury? Would Joel have been less severely disabled and more physically self-sufficient if IL services had been available to him immediately after he completed his active medical rehabilitation process? It is impossible to be certain of what the results would have been, but it is probable that his condition would not have deteriorated as much as it did.

## IMPROVING COMMUNITY-BASED MEDICAL CARE

One method by which community-based medical care for disabled persons could be improved involves basic alterations in the way medical students are ti..ined. First, all medical students should be required to take courses in physical medicine and rehabilitation, thus exposing them to the rehabilitation model of medical treatment. Second, in order to combat the current image of physical medicine and rehabilitation as a speciality that is both unrewarding and uninteresting, medical students should be made aware of the major role technology plays in the field, which is on the leading edge of medical advances.

The burgeoning of biomedical advances has resulted in even the most profoundly disabled person being able to function more independently to some degree, which gives medical practitioners in the field a greater sense of accomplishment than they may have had previously. The recent wedding between the fields of medicine and engineering has resulted in a new rehabilitation-related discipline, rehabilitation engineering. Rehabilitation engineering uses lasers, microelectrodes, and microcomputers to enhance the physical function and communication skills of people who formerly would have remained totally physically dependent and unable to communicate. Moreover, in areas with rehabilitation engineering clinics, personnel are available to consult with general medical practitioners on possible treatment techniques for people with a variety of disabling conditions.

With the advent of treatment innovations in the field of rehabilitation medicine, it may be possible to alter the traditional cause-result-treatment-cure orientation of medicine so that medical success can be defined not only as total physical restoration, but also as total role restoration, whether or not any physical limitations remain. If success for medical treatment were redefined, the incorporation of medical rehabilitation practices into the practice of general medicine would result in increased satisfaction for those who treat disabled people. Anthropologists point out that what best distinguishes man from his fellow creatures is his ability to devise and use tools to control and modify his environment. In terms of innate strength and physical dexterity man will always be inferior. It could be argued that man's greatest achievement, therefore, could be the development of technology and the transfer of that technology into devices that permit people with severe physical impairments to, nonetheless, control their own lives and master their environments.

Medical care for the disabled could also be improved by a revision of the techniques of teaching medical self-management to disabled people. While patient education has always been a prescribed part of the overall rehabilitation process, the thoroughness and timing of patient education has sometimes been less than ideal. As part of their medical rehabilitation, for example, VA hospitals with spinal cord injury units offer patients classes covering every aspect of medical self-management, from catheter and skin care to dealing with autonomic dysreflexia. As part of the educational effort, pamphlets are distributed to new patients to explain what a spinal cord injury is, what services the VA offers to spinal cord injured patients, and what the recommended techniques for detecting and preventing common complications of spinal cord injury are.

Too often, however, efforts to educate patients are more effective in concept than in reality. More time and effort may be devoted to the creation and distribution of educational materials than to ensuring that patients use and understand the materials they are given. Many of the pamphlets that are intended to enhance patients' ability to deal with the health care aspects of their disabilities are written at too high a level for many patients to understand. In addition, these educational materials tend to be distributed to patients as soon as they have been admitted for treatment, long before they are able to see the relevance of the information to their own situations. Even when patients read the information, they often forget it because it is too soon for them to put that information to practical use. The medical rehabilitation team, however, with many other responsibilities to contend with, often assumes that discharged patients are more knowledgeable in health care matters than is, in fact, the case.

Craig Rehabilitation Hospital, a civilian spinal cord injury center near Denver, has compiled a manual on the sexual functioning of men and women with spinal cord injury and the effects of such an injury on a person's sexuality. The Craig manual is an outstanding example of educational materials that are well designed to meet the needs of the various kinds of people who share a specific disability. Written in a readable, nonthreatening style, this manual, as well as covering all the physical consequences of a spinal cord injury, explores in depth the interpersonal aspects of an intimate relationship when one partner in the relationship has a cord injury.

Even with the best-designed patient education program, however, some people will not be able to master the necessary health care information and techniques during the brief time they are actively engaged in the medical rehabilitation process. Those who are in the second stage of denial (see Chapter 5) still believe that they will recover completely, and so conclude they have no need to learn health care techniques specific to their disabling condition. Others may not be concerned about or may actually welcome the possibility of acquiring additional medical problems, due to a not uncommon aberration that sometimes stems from prolonged hospitalization. Fearful of being expelled from the security of a specialized environment where they are confident that their physical needs will be met, patients who are about to be discharged sometimes try to catch a cold or create a self-inflicted skin lesion, which would allow them to prolong their hospitalization. In short, some newly disabled people will not reach the degree of psychological adjustment that they need in order to benefit fully from educational efforts concerning the function of their bodies or medical self-management.

To ensure that any educational gains made will not be lost because of patients' misunderstanding or unwillingness to accept responsibility for their own physical wellbeing, rehabilitation facilities also conduct medical education programs for patients' families. These programs tend to vary in content and intensity from one rehabilitation facility to the next.

When polio was epidemic, family members of patients at the Georgia Warm Springs Foundation would spend three to four days at the foundation being trained in techniques for taking care of and assisting people severely disabled by polio. If patients were able to dress themselves, their relatives were taught not to help them dress, but if they were unable to dress without assistance, then relatives were taught how best to provide whatever assistance was needed. During this time the Polio Foundation was well funded and was able to cover the expenses of family members who traveled to Warm Springs for specialized training.

Today, education of family members is still considered to be an important part of the rehabilitation process, but the cost of such efforts has increased substantially, while available funds have decreased. Today, in most facilities, before patients who are not self-sufficient are discharged, the person or persons who will be assisting them may spend one day in the facility to become familiar with a specific individual's routine over a 24-hour period. The limited time allotted to family education tends to slant that education toward techniques for helping, rather than toward developing the sense of discrimination to determine when assistance is necessary and when it is not.

## ROLE OF IL SERVICES IN COMMUNITY-BASED MEDICAL CARE

IL programs are not designed to provide medical treatment to disabled people. Provision of direct medical services would not only replicate services that, theoretically, already exist, but would also require increased funding and staffing of IL programs. Moreover, incorporating medical treatment into IL programs would lessen their overall effectiveness by turning them into extensions of the medical model of treatment, instead of allowing them to offer a rehabilitation model based on a community-living orientation and emphasizing the nonphysical factors involved in functional independence.

IL services have, as one of their objectives, the promotion of appropriate and adequate health care for program recipients. The role of IL programs, in this respect, is (1) to make existing medical services more accessible to disabled people; (2) to enhance their health maintenance skills; (3) to supplement the health education they acquired as part of their intensive medical rehabilitation; and (4) to monitor their health care needs.

Several factors that affect the health care needs of disabled people have been identified. According to Kaplan (1979), readmission to acute care hospitals is related to (1) client income; (2) marital status; and (3) degree of community integration. People with adequate incomes, who are married, or who actively participate in community activities, are less likely to develop illnesses severe enough to require hospitalization, while type and severity of disability is unrelated to the need for health care.

IL programs whose main purpose is to promote greater community integration are, therefore, directly concerned with the health care needs of those they serve. In cases like Joel's, IL services can be geared to arrange for retraining in ADL. Programs that have on staff either an occupational therapist or a counselor who specializes in teaching IL skills may provide this retraining directly. Other programs may have to arrange for the parttime services of a trained professional either directly or under the sponsorship of a rehabilitation agency, such as the Division of Vocational Rehabilitation (DVR), when job placement is considered a possibility.

Many IL centers have developed training modules (short, intensive courses in areas important to independent functioning), one of which will teach clients normal body functioning, the effects of their disabilities on body functioning, and the proper use and care of the body. Such a medical module, specifically tailored for Joel, would have included techniques for properly padding portions of the body most vulnerable to pressure sores, for checking for and identifying early signs of skin breakdown, and for maintaining a free and copious drainage of urine to prevent urinary infections and the development of kidney and bladder stones. While much of the information contained within a medical module may have been covered while a person was actively engaged in medical rehabilitation, as with Joel, some people may not have mastered or put into practice the skills they were once taught. In some instances, however, the medical problems disabled people experience may be unavoidable, for even the most health conscious cannot always avoid becoming ill, sometimes seriously.

As part of their peer counseling services, IL programs provide counselors who can act as medical role models to demonstrate methods of medical self-management that will not only help clients prevent unnecessary medical complications from developing, but will demonstrate to them the way to cope with problems that do arise. Clients must accept the fact that they must monitor their bodies' functioning for the rest of their lives, if they are to maintain an optimum level of functioning.

Monitoring of clients' health care needs must concern itself with the side-effects and interactions of medications taken for chronic health problems. To teach clients self-monitoring skills, programs should include in their resources standard references, such as the *Physicians' Desk Reference* (PDR), which clients can use to routinely check on any medications that are prescribed for them. In addition to teaching clients how to utilize such references, programs should also train clients to become more assertive in their interactions with physicians regarding the ramifications of particular medications for people with their specific disabilities. For example, people with impaired respiratory functioning, such as respiratory postpolios or people with advanced emphysema, should not take certain pain medications or muscle relaxants that may reduce their ability to move air in and out of their lungs, thus precipitating a respiratory crisis.

When receiving community-based medical treatment, people who have a solid understanding of their own physical conditions will be aware of proper treatment procedures when they seek treatment for any acute illness. If their primary care physician is unaware of the potentially serious consequences of following otherwise normal treatment procedures, they themselves must know enough to ask the appropriate questions in an appropriate manner, so that the physician will be willing to double-check any treatment he or she provides.

Finally, an IL program can increase the availability of community medical services by acting as an advocate for accessibility in transportation and treatment sites, by educating the community about the health care needs of disabled people and by providing information and referral services regarding available community health care. Programs that establish good relationships with medical treatment facilities can fill an essential role as a health care liaison between members of the general medical community and people whose very existence may depend on the quality and availability of the health care services they require.

# 7

## Essential Home Services— Home, Health, and Personal Maintenance

If severely disabled people of any age are to live outside of custodial institutions, certain essential home services must be available to them. The three categories of home services that are required for people with severe physical limitations are those that provide (1) supplementary housekeeping services, such as cleaning, meal preparation and yard maintenance; (2) supplementary medical and nursing care; and (3) assistance in carrying out daily self-care routines, such as bathing, dressing, or toileting. Without these services many severely disabled people cannot live within the community with safety and convenience.

Early in the spring of 1982 the bodies of two wealthy sisters were discovered in their high-rise New York apartment, approximately three months after the first had died. The one who died first had had a fatal heart attack. The other, who was severely disabled and who required her sister's assistance to meet all her personal needs, died of "natural causes" several days afterwards. Their bodies were discovered by a marshal who had come to evict them because they hadn't been paying their rent.

**129**

Some months earlier two items appeared in the news media concerning elderly disabled people. The first described the ordeal of a woman who had remained trapped in her bathtub for two days. Unable to get out of the tub after she had finished bathing, she kept warm by periodically running hot water into the tub and covering herself with bathtowels. Eventually, a neighbor who came to visit discovered her predicament and rescued her. The second involved a woman who also lived by herself. One evening when she was cleaning up her kitchen, she backed into a large waste basket, lost her balance, and fell into it. Unable to extricate herself, she remained trapped in the wastebasket until her son, worried because she was not answering her telephone, found her.

These three stories illustrate not only the vital need that severely disabled people have for home services, but also three underlying facts concerning home services for the disabled. First, adequate financial resources, by themselves, cannot competely shield disabled people from harm or bodily neglect. Second, some category of home services is essential for any severely disabled person who wants to live within the community. Third, home services, which on the surface appear to meet only specific home, health, or personal maintenance needs, actually provide much more: they provide the structure and interpersonal contacts that are vitally necessary to the physical and psychological wellbeing of severely disabled people.

Rather than serving as a protection against the vicissitudes of advanced age or a lack of physical strength and dexterity, in certain situations being financially independent can prevent a person in desperate need of certain services from receiving them. Social service workers in large metropolitan areas encounter many instances where publicly supported, life-sustaining or life-enhancing services are unavailable to people who do not live in impoverished areas. For example, meals-on-wheels services are often unavailable in affluent neighborhoods, because these neighborhoods usually lie outside clearly defined service catchment areas. Moreover, privately supported social services, too, are only available within impoverished areas and to people with limited financial resources.

Unless a disabled person who lives in an affluent neighborhood has friends and family who live nearby, he or she may live an isolated life in the midst of unconcerned, often transient neighbors. The situation may be compounded by the fact that the person is unused to contacting and seeking help from social service organizations and agencies. Pride may make the person reluctant to admit to anyone that his or her living situation is potentially dangerous because a hearing impairment makes it difficult to use a telephone, a visual impairment makes it impossible to drive, or a mobility impairment prevents the use of what public transportation may be available.

Irrespective of the financial status of severely disabled people in the community, certain home services play a vital role. For the indigent and the affluent alike, most of the problems associated with obtaining essential home services are identical: defining what services are indispensable; deciding the extent and the scheduling of needed services; and discovering a reliable source to provide those services. The one major difference is that once these shared problems have been solved, the indigent still face the problem of finding a third-party payer who can authorize the provision of needed services, while the affluent can underwrite the costs of needed services themselves.

The chapter will

1. describe the types of home services that most disabled individuals require,

2. explain how personal care attendants (PCAs) contribute to the success of IL efforts,

3. discuss the recruitment, training, and retention of PCAs,

4. discuss the role of IL programs in the provision of essential home services.

## CATEGORIES OF HOME SERVICES ESSENTIAL TO INDEPENDENT LIVING

Without some type of financial assistance, few disabled people could afford the kinds and variety of home services that would make it possible for them to live within the community. Before public support for the necessary funding can be elicited, however, the feasibility of such services must be demonstrated. It must be shown that providing these services in a community setting improves the quality of disabled people's lives and reduces or, at least, does not exceed the cost of providing life-sustaining and income maintenance services to disabled people in institutional or custodial settings.

Although the concept of independent living is not supported by all disabled people (Goldenson et al., 1978; Laurie, 1977) and life in the community may result in fewer social interactions than life in an institution (Berkson and Romer, 1981; Knight, 1980), objections to the concept stem primarily from a misunderstanding of IL goals and services. Fully implemented, IL services will not place disabled people in physical jeopardy or under insupportable psychological stress (DeLoach and Greer, 1981; Heal, Sigelman, and Switzky, 1980). Moreover, fully implemented IL services will extend and enhance individuals' interpersonal relationships (Edgerton and Bercovici, 1976). As Berkson and Romer (1981) point out, being in daily contact with staff members and fellow residents within an institutional setting leads to a greater number of interpersonal contacts, but also to residents being treated like children. In such settings, disabled people experience a nearly total lack of privacy and are unable to choose the people with whom they associate.

The type and number of home services necessary to sustain a person within the community will vary with the nature of the disability, the personality and emotional stability, and the age of the person in question. Apart from differences that result from interpersonal variables, however, the various types of home services that are required by severely disabled people can be divided into three overlapping categories: health care services, home care services, and personal care services.

## HOME HEALTH CARE SERVICES

The current health care system in our society is biased toward placing disabled people in hospitals or nursing homes, although the rising costs of health care are beginning to change that bias. For example, prior to 1981 Medicare did not pay for a substantial number of home health care services. Only if an individual were in a nursing home or institution would Medicare cover 100 percent of health care costs. For disabled people who were employed or for disabled children who lived at home with their parents, Medicare paid nothing at all.

Then, in 1981, Medicaid Section 21 was passed as part of the Omnibus Reconciliation Act of 1981. Medicaid 21, as it is called, gives states the option of providing a variety of home health services with Medicaid funds. The rationale for this change in policy is contained within the wording of Medicaid 21: "Many elderly, disabled and chronically ill persons live in institutions not for medical reasons, but because of the paucity of health and social services in their communities, and their inability to pay for those services or to have them covered by Medicaid when they do exist." According to Shaw (1981), "Supporters of Medicaid Section 21 intend that a wide variety of non-institutional services be covered."

In the language of Section 21, "Often such services can be provided most efficiently and effectively by professionals other than physicians, such as social workers and nurses, qualified mental retardation professionals, and by non-professionals, such as nurses aides, homemakers and personal care attendants." If states choose to implement their Medicaid option, they may provide respite care services to families with disabled adults or children, as well as day care services for adults. Moreover, the provision of aid to qualified individuals for nursing services, medical supplies and equipment, physical and occupational therapy, speech pathology and audiology is covered under Section 21.

If Eleanor had been eligible under Section 21, following the surgery to replace her degenerated hip joint she would have been able to benefit from the nursing, physical therapy, and homemaking services. These services would have allowed her to avoid an extended and expensive stay in the nursing home. Several conditions must be met, however, which can preclude the provision of home health care services in certain cases. First, each case has to be reviewed by a preassessment team (PAT) to determine whether a person would benefit more from institutionalization than from living within the community. Second, evidence must be presented to the Secretary of Health and Human Services that more Medicaid funds are not being spent on providing home health care services than would be spent if health care services were being provided in an institutional setting.

Even when Medicaid funds are not involved, as when a private insurance carrier is paying for health care services, the acceleration of medical costs has caused the home health care industry to flourish. Kidney dialysis, whether hemodialysis or peritoneal dialysis, is less expensive and less disruptive to a person's daily routine when carried out at home, rather than in a medical setting. Similarly, people with advanced emphysema or with severe asthmatic or cardiac conditions can now receive the oxygen therapy they require at home. Moreover, if their conditions allow them to make use of the lightweight, portable oxygen packs that are now available, they can move freely about their communities without risking their physical well-being. People who are dependent on respiratory aids, such as a rocking bed, or a tank or chest respirator, are able to use these aids in a home setting, which allows them to maintain more normal lifestyles. Finally, people with urinary diversions, ileostomies, or colostomies who for some reason are unable to manage the care of their own devices find the services of visiting nurses or home health aides to be invaluable in keeping these devices functioning properly, thus preventing potentially costly complications.

Whether they are catheter-changing services from a home health aide, gait training from a physical therapist, or breathing exercises from a respiration therapist, home health services are an essential component of IL services. First, these services can make the difference between individuals living comfortably and safely at home or remaining in a more specialized, and therefore more expensive, medical setting. Second, as discussed in Chapter 6, home health services can prevent the development of new disabling conditions or the exacerbation of existing chronic conditions. With home health care services, severely disabled individuals of any age are likely to lose their functional skills less rapidly than they otherwise might.

## HOME MAINTENANCE SERVICES

One of the first questions that arises when disabled people consider buying or returning to a single-family dwelling is how they will manage basic home maintenance chores. Rising material and labor costs place an increasingly insupportable financial burden even on people who can effect minor home repairs and alterations without assistance. For those who lack manual strength and dexterity or who cannot use a stepstool or ladder safely, even such minor housekeeping tasks as changing a light bulb are difficult. For more severely disabled people, they are impossible.

Fortunately, many home maintenance chores that require little time, effort, or skill can be delayed until a friend, neighbor, or door-to-door salesman arrives who is able and willing to tighten a loose screw, retrieve an object from a hard-to-reach storage area, or replace a light bulb. In her book *You Can Do It from a Wheelchair* (1973) Gilbert suggests that mobility-impaired people leave tasks like washing windows or watering hanging plants for a more able spouse or child. Fay S., a medical secretary who is in a wheelchair, maintains her own apartment, including cleaning, except she routinely has friends whom she has invited for dinner dust the top of the refrigerator. With this exception, everything in her home, including kitchen storage areas, was specially constructed at a more convenient height.

Careful placement and selection of household items, deliberate installation of pulleys that allow hanging lamps to be lowered when bulbs need replacing, and agreements with salesmen that heavy pieces of furniture will have casters added before a purchase is finalized help circumvent some home maintenance problems. More difficult to manage, however, are the many major home maintenance tasks that, if neglected, can create even more extensive and expensive problems, including structural damage to one's home. Plumbing, appliance, and electrical repairs make up the bulk of the indoor home maintenance tasks that are beyond the capabilities of most severely disabled adults.

Maintenance problems affecting the exterior of a home tend to occur less frequently, but also tend to be more expensive to correct. Peeling paint, plugged-up rain gutters, crumbling concrete foundations or ramps, and leaking roofs are serious in themselves, to say nothing of the additional problems each can precipitate. Disabled people who live in single family dwellings must also make arrangements to maintain the lawn and yard. In the summer, grass must be mowed frequently. In the spring and fall, leaves and fallen branches must be raked, bagged, and carried away. In the winter, driveways and sidewalks must be cleared of snow and ice. And throughout the year, the branches of trees and shrubs that could damage the roof or siding must be pruned.

Many disabled people are overwhelmed by the potential problems associated with living in a house of their own and decide to live in a condominium or apartment, instead. For those who prefer to live in a privately owned house, however, there are ways to minimize home maintenance problems, but only with the expenditure of a great deal of thought or money or both. For example, people with adequate incomes can employ a yardman or contract for the services of a professional lawn care company. People with limited incomes can contact church groups, high schools, or senior citizens centers to find young people or retirees who will do yard work inexpensively. As a public service in the spring, many daily newspapers run a special edition of free classified advertisements for teenagers who need summer employment. Typically, the odd jobs these teenagers are willing to perform range from grooming family pets to planting trees and shrubs. Then too, many people with disabilities who have home maintenance skills prefer these kinds of jobs because they can work the hours and at the pace they choose, which is especially important for those who experience fatigue as a side-effect of their disabling condition.

A final option open to some disabled people is to develop a method that allows them to carry out routine maintenance tasks themselves, so that the need for assistance is reduced to only the more demanding household chores. For example, a few mechanically minded people have devised remote control systems that allow them to operate power lawmowers from a distance. Such systems work well only on small, level, grassy plots where no trees or shrubs block the path of the mower. Even here there is always the possibility that a bit of debris or thatch will cause the mower to stall, creating a need for someone to approach the mower and remove whatever is interfering with its operation.

Others use ground covers, such as ivy or vicuna, which eventually eliminate grass and weeds from a lawn and do not require mowing. When a yard is small, grass can be replaced with a pine bark mulch if the yard is not going to be used. Disabled people who enjoy gardening and who can afford it may have their lawns replaced with washed concrete and have large tubs or built-up planters installed, which will both reduce the need for yard work and allow them to grow flowers or vegetables (Hale, 1979). For many, however, washed concrete and specially constructed planters will be prohibitively expensive. These people will find that large sheets of black plastic will eliminate the problems of lawn maintenance when spread over the yard and, with slits cut in them for plants, will provide a virtually weed-free gardening area. Hale (1979) offers several designs for outdoor modifications, such as hard-surfaced yards and wooden decks, that can allow people with the most severely disabling conditions the enjoyment of gardening.

Whichever option disabled people choose, they will be unable to avoid altogether the need for assistance and for incurring some expense, at least initially. Friends or relatives can reduce the overall cost of modifying a yard. Often such people are eager to devote themselves to a project that requires a one-time expenditure on their part. When those who are close to someone who has had a disabling accident or illness feel thwarted because they can do nothing to help restore his or her lost physical capabilities, they may welcome the opportunity to do anything that has a tangible benefit for the disabled person.

Unfortunately, home maintenance services that involve yard work or the repair and upkeep of a building or appliances are not considered to be vital to the wellbeing of disabled people. Such services, therefore, are not covered under Section 21, nor are expenses for such services allowed as either a medical or a child-care/homemaker deduction by the Internal Revenue Service.

Finally, included within the general category of home maintenance services are homemaker services, which are covered under Medicaid if they are determined to fill a home health care need. The cost of homemaker services is also considered a legitimate income tax deduction if the presence of a homemaker, in a situation where one spouse is severely disabled, allows the other spouse to be remuneratively employed. Ironically, when the husband and wife are both severely disabled and employed, with their continued employment dependent upon their receiving assistance with cleaning, laundry, and meal preparation, no such deduction is allowed.

Homemaking services can be obtained in one of two ways. First, a person may be employed on a regular basis to come into the home once a day, once a week, or somewhere in between, to clean and keep the mechanics of the home running smoothly. Most valuable is the kind of homemaker who not only cleans and does the laundry but who also alerts the employer when appliances are not working properly and when cleaning materials need to be replaced, and who keeps the linens sorted and clothes in good repair.

Second, homemaking services can be obtained through a contract with a company that employs, trains, and supervises cleaning crews that descend on a home for several hours to wash and wax floors, change bedding, and clean kitchens and bathrooms in what Europeans call a "blitz" clean. Typically, professional housecleaning companies provide heavy housecleaning as well as light housecleaning services, but do not provide the personal touches that are invaluable to severely disabled people. For example, packing and storing away Christmas decorations or placing houseplants outdoors in spring and bringing them indoors in the fall are not the kinds of services usually provided by a professional cleaning company. Nevertheless, these kinds of personal services are often among those most needed by disabled individuals who want to live as "normal" a life as possible.

Disabled people, like people in general, find homemakers through newspaper ads, through the recommendations of friends, and through employment agencies. For those who require homemakers with a special understanding of their physical requirements, some religious denominations operate training and placement services for homemakers who, for the minimum wage, will provide personal care services. These church-sponsored homemaking services, which are primarily designed to provide jobs for needy parishioners and to provide a source of temporary help for people recovering from acute illnesses, can be of particular benefit to those who require reliable help on a long-term basis.

## PERSONAL CARE SERVICES

Personal care services are those services that are designed to assist disabled people with their personal maintenance requirements: bathing, dressing, toileting, and grooming. In some cases they are considered home health services, and so are often covered by Medicaid and private insurance carriers. Where they differ from health services is in the degree of medical skill or knowledge required of the care provider. For example, home health services are primarily designed to help a person recover from a decubitus ulcer, regain strength after a heart attack, or cope with a home dialysis program. Personal care services tend to be more preventative in nature and may consist of irrigating and changing catheters and assisting with toileting to prevent infections or impactions, or maintaining good hygiene and checking the skin daily to prevent skin breakdowns from occurring.

It has been claimed that good personal care services and personal care attendants (PCAs) are the key to successful independent living, at least for people who can never attain total physical self-sufficiency. The remainder of this chapter will be devoted to the PCAs, because without them independent living, as a service paradigm, could not achieve its full potential.

## ATTENDANT SERVICES: THE KEY TO SUCCESS

The very concept of the PCA embodies the basic difference between the IL paradigm and the medical model of rehabilitation. As DeJong and Wenkler (1979) point out, the self-directed nature of a situation where the disabled person solicits and controls the care rendered to him by a PCA encapsulates the philosophy of independent living in a clearly defined, person-to-person, direct service. For example, the home health services, which were discussed above, are based on the medical model. In this model a nurse or homemaker is paid by a third party—an insurance company, Medicare, or Medicaid—to enter the home of a disabled person to provide services that have been prescribed by someone other than the person needing them. Under this model, the employee is recruited, trained, paid, and supervised through a system established and controlled by the third party payer. Moreover, the exact nature and scope of the services for which the disabled person is eligible are also determined by the agency or company that provides the funds.

Attendant care in the IL model differs significantly from attendant care in the medical model, although the nature and scope of the services rendered may be identical. In the IL model, the disabled person decides who is hired to work as a PCA, when a PCA is terminated and exactly what a PCA's duties are. Even when public monies pay for the services of a PCA, those monies go first to the disabled person, who then uses them to pay the PCA.

This subtle, but all-important shifting of the locus of control increases the disabled individual's authority and status as a psychologically competent human being, both from his or her own point of view and from that of the PCA. Under the medical model, where treatment decisions are arrived at and implemented by someone else, a disabled person is cast into much the same role as a family pet—vitally concerned with, but powerless to influence, daily health and personal care routines.

According to DeJong and Wenkler (1979), approximately 1.1 percent of people between the ages of 16 and 65 and approximately 6.5 percent of elderly people require some assistance with their daily activities. This need for assistance can have a devastating effect on their confidence in their abilit y to control and direct their own lives. While self-care activities are the first activities that humans are taught and expected to carry out independently, they are the last activities in which people who acquire disabilities regain full independence. In the IL paradigm, despite the fact that disabled individuals may need to rely on someone else for their most intimate physiological needs, they can maintain their sense of personal autonomy because they retain basic control over the management of those needs.

## PROBLEMS IN OBTAINING ATTENDANT CARE

Unfortunately, while for many severely disabled people attendant care is the key to successful independent living, satisfactory attendant care services are often difficult to obtain. Several major problems face those in need of assistance with their personal care: funding for PCA services and recruitment and retention of qualified PCAs. The problem with retention is often associated with severely disabled persons, who may have difficulty relating to PCAs.

**Funding** Employee dissatisfaction and high turnover, stemming largely from unacceptable salary levels, underlie all the problems related to implementing attendant care services satisfactorily. Depending on the area where a disabled person lives, salaries for PCAs range from the minimum wage to $6.00 an hour. Since disabled people require anywhere from 2 to 24 hours of attendant care per day, few can afford the attendant services they require unless they receive some supplementary financial assistance. People's eligibility for financial assistance is, in turn, dependent on their being eligible for some type of publicly funded, income maintenance benefits. For example, availability of funds for PCAs under Medicaid is limited to those who are eligible for SSI payments.

In Massachusetts, IL centers such as the Boston Center for Independent Living, have contracts with the state Medicaid to provide attendant care and housekeeping services to those whom the public welfare department has determined to be eligible. In Minnesota, the state Medicaid funds attendant care directly, without the intervention of the local IL centers. Unlike those in Massachusetts, housekeeping services are covered under the Title XX program.

Under Title XX of the Social Security Act, payments for PCAs are allowed without the medical provisions of the Medicaid program. According to DeJong and Wenkler (1979), the California attendant care program is administered by the county departments of public welfare. The number of hours of assistance required is determined by a social worker, based on a client interview and a physician's statement that attendant care is required. Once the need and the amount of time are established, the client, who is reimbursed for each hour allotted at a rate equal to the current minimum wage, arranges and pays for his or her own attendant care.

Unfortunately, under both Title XX and Medicaid, a person will become ineligible for attendant benefits if he or she becomes gainfully employed. Most jobs, however, do not pay enough to cover both the costs of employment and the cost of an attendant whose services are essential if the person is to retain the job. Since the requirements that govern a person's eligibility to acquire the monies to retain a PCA undermine the very principles on which IL goals are based, it may be necessary to abolish the link between a proven need for income assistance and eligibility for funding. In DeJong's opinion, "attendant care should be an entitlement service that is related to a person's functional capacity," not to his or her vocational status.

**Recruitment and Retention**   In theory, attendant care epitomizes the IL paradigm by shifting control of the attendant-attendee relationship from the care provider, via the third party payer, to the person who requires the care. In actuality, however, the difficulties inherent in recruiting, training, retaining and paying a PCA who is both reliable and competent lessen the amount of control that disabled people can exercise.

Most laypeople, including attendants, find it difficult to accept that people who are unable to carry out the most basic self-care tasks themselves can, nevertheless, competently schedule and direct the carrying out of these tasks by someone else. In order to live a self-governing life, disabled people must maintain their authority, and their ability to do so is threatened by these doubts on the part of others. When those others are PCAs, on whom disabled people must rely for their continued existence, that threat is compounded. Physically dependent people often find themselves in the position of having to choose between exercising control at the risk of alienating or losing their attendants and relinquishing that control to ensure their physical security.

The dilemma that many severely disabled people find themselves in stems from the difficulties they encounter in trying to locate and then retain competent PCAs. According to Smith (1977), the prospect of a minimum wage attracts few qualified people into a job that is demanding in terms of both responsibility and time. Although for most PCAs the actual time spent performing specified tasks is relatively brief—the average range is from two to four hours a day—the time during which they must be available in case their assistance is required can be 24 hours a day. As a result, many of those attracted to attendant work are "marginal in mental or emotional stability, intelligence or competence" (Smith and Meyer, 1981).

Although finding qualified attendants is difficult, a variety of recruitment methods have proved successful for some people some of the time—placing job advertisements in newspapers and church bulletins; posting ads on bulletin boards in public libraries, grocery stores, college dormitories, and student religious centers; recruiting people who are already employed in minimum-wage jobs in nursing homes, hospitals and restaurants; contacting job banks that handle applications from retirees and high-school or college students; and contacting IL programs that maintain registries of people who are willing to work as PCAs. Smith (1977) recommends recruiting college students as attendants. According to Smith, jobs with intermittent periods of idle time, as PCA jobs tend to be, are well tailored for college students' need for income and intermittent studying time. Smith also cites instances in which the pairing of a physically disabled person with a mentally retarded person has worked well in meeting the independent living needs of both. The mentally retarded person can contribute needed physical strength and dexterity to the relationship and the physically disabled person financial and social judgment. Finally, Smith suggests recruiting aliens as attendants. Aliens may be willing to work for a minimum wage if they are provided with the security of a home while they are learning to cope within the American culture.

Unfortunately, those who are most readily available to work as PCAs are also the people least likely to remain in the job for an extended period. The average length of employment for a PCA is six months (Smith and Meyer, 1981), although PCAs have remained working for the same person for as short a time as two hours and for as long a time as 24 years. The following factors have been identified as contributing to the low job satisfaction and consequent high turnover of PCAs: low wages; lack of fringe benefits; low job status; responsibility for the physical wellbeing and, in some cases, the life of the employer; and the nature of the duties involved.

POTENTIAL SOLUTIONS

Job satisfaction is not entirely absent among PCAs (Smith and Meyer, 1981), and several measures can be taken to help enhance recruitment and retention efforts. The intervention of an IL program in the recruitment of PCAs and in the training of both PCAs and their potential employers has proven to ameliorate the problems a solitary potential PCA employer faces.

For example, some IL programs have launched successful PCA recruitment and training programs that establish a link between those who want to employ a PCA and those who are willing to seek this type of employment. While IL programs utilize the same recruitment procedures listed above, in addition they often work with people in vocational education centers where potential PCAs can be trained. Then the IL programs maintain lists of specially trained attendants that clients can consult when they require the services of a PCA on a short-term basis, as well as when they seek fulltime attendant care.

IL programs also work directly with clients. Program staff may train disabled people in how to interview applicants for a position, in how to provide exact job descriptions to potential employees, and in how to fire an unsatisfactory attendant. IL programs can also assist by helping to coordinate the personal care needs of several clients with the employment needs of several PCAs. By sharing attendant services, clients collectively can often pay a more attractive salary. By sharing attendees, PCAs can often schedule their duties so they have more free time and more flexible working hours. Moreover, the resultant increase in job satisfaction may do more than reduce the high turnover rate among PCAs in general. It may also enhance future recruitment efforts as more potential PCAs become aware that this type of employment allows high-school and college students to earn a salary while receiving their room and board and allows older people to supplement their retirement incomes while eliminating their need to maintain a home of their own.

By providing services to those in need of a PCA, IL programs can foster their clients' motivation to live more independently. In order for severely disabled people to willingly assume the risks inherent in an independent lifestyle, they need assurance that they will not have to deal with potentially life-threatening situations alone (see Chapter 11). They have to be confident that, if an attendant proves to be unreliable, a system of IL services exists that will ensure that they will not suffer the fate of the woman in New York, who died because the assistance she needed was no longer available.

# 8

## Independent Living
## and a Barrier-Free Environment

The relationship between being able to have an independent life-style and a barrier-free environment is clear. Without the absence of manmade barriers in architecture and various modes of public and private transportation, severely disabled people cannot exercise the mobility necessary for them to function at their optimum levels of independence. The effectiveness of IL programs depends, therefore, on the pre-existence or the continual evolution of barrier-free environments. Without accessible homes, workplaces, public buildings, and businesses, without accessible and affordable means of transportation, independent living is an inoperable service concept, doomed to fail because of seemingly insurmountable but socially remediable environmental factors. Without the elimination of manmade obstacles, severely disabled people, in general, will remain in an unnecessary state of dependency.

One of the most damaging misconceptions concerning the social impact of barrier-free design is that proposed design changes will benefit only people with the most visible mobility impairments—those who use wheelchairs. But wheelchair users comprise only a small percentage of the approximately 17.5 million people who cannot used conventionally designed public conveyances or who cannot enter unassisted the majority of public and privately owned buildings constructed before the early 1970s.

One middle-aged member of the larger, hidden minority is a woman with Parkinson's disease who lives in a quiet neighborhood near the center of a large Southern city. Although this woman takes daily strolls that take her farther than the three city blocks between her home and the nearest bus stop, she cannot ride the city's buses because she cannot safely mount the steps of a conventionally designed bus. This woman's mobility is also limited within the neighborhood in which she lives. A naturally gregarious person, she has limited social contacts with her neighbors because none have homes with low or ramped entrances that would allow her to enter safely and conveniently. Yet, to any stranger who passes her on the street, she appears to be an ordinary woman, albeit with somewhat poor posture, who is taking a leisurely walk. Nevertheless, she and millions like her are totally disenfranchised when it comes to being able to use transportation supposedly designed to serve the public or being able to go where they choose, because of the limitations imposed by outmoded architectural designs.

The term "architectural modification," which is often used interchangeably with "barrier-removal" or "barrier-free" design, is in itself misleading. It implies that there is a normal way to design buildings or transportation systems and that only by violating these normal modes of design can people with mobility impairments gain access to their communities. Bowe (1978) has pointed out that if accessibility features had been incorporated into buildings and transportation systems as soon as any once-valid reasons for flights of stairs and high-floored conveyances had ceased to exist, barrier-free design would be the accepted mode of design, instead of the controversial issue it too often is now. Once, long flights of stairs, like the poles that elevate homes in rural tropical areas, afforded home dwellers protection against invaders, animal or human. Fortress cities, like Mont Saint Michel, were built on as high a vantage point as possible, with several internal walls or levels, each more militarily secure than the one before. But while modern warfare has rendered the depths of the earth a safer haven than the peaks of mountains, a cultural lag exists between designs that are practical and designs that are viewed as aesthetically pleasing. The steps of the Capitol Building in Washington, D.C., convey a sense of power and majesty but do nothing to conserve the energies of people who need to enter the building several times a day. Until the convenience of the general public becomes the determining factor in the design and layout of all types of structures, from federal buildings to private homes, many people will be adversely affected, and not only those with mobility impairments.

Barrier-free design is convenient for everyone, the young and the elderly, people moving furniture and people with children in strollers. For physically disabled people, however, barrier-free design is more than a convenience. For those with mobility impairments, a barrier-free environment is a necessity that not only falls within the same category of basic needs as food and shelter, but is a prerequisite for obtaining all other basic needs.

This chapter will

1. review legislation that was drafted in order to promote a barrier-free environment,

2. relate the three levels of independence, which were introduced in Chapter 2, to accessibility features within homes and communities,

3. discuss the advantages and disadvantages of modifying existing buildings and transportation systems, as opposed to mandating accessibility in new construction and new public conveyances,

4. demonstrate the importance of barrier-free design to independent living.

## ENVIRONMENTAL BARRIERS TO SUCCESSFUL REHABILITATION

In retrospect, the advances in barrier removal in the middle and late 1970s stemmed more from the efforts of disabled activists and their advocates in the rehabilitation professions than from the response of the general public to a concrete social need. Before the 1970s there was no coordinated national effort to accommodate the increasing numbers of people who could not use existing buildings and public transportation services. During this early period, when mobility-impaired people did gain entrance to museums, restaurants, schools, or businesses without assistance, it was usually because a rear entrance was at ground level or a ramp existed for the convenience of employees in moving heavy items. When it came to public transportation, however, alternative accessible entrances did not exist, and few disabled people were able to travel around enough to make use of what accessible elevators and back entrances there were. The lack of overall accessibility, and consequent absence of mobility-impaired people in public places, helped perpetuate negative social attitudes concerning the disabled. These attitudes questioned not only the desirability of having disabled people participate in community activities, but also the need for barrier-free design. Many people questioned the advisability of barrier-removal efforts, since few severely disabled people were ever seen in public.

Social attitudes are of paramount importance in understanding the attitudinal barriers that result in the lack of needed services to disabled people. They have been the subject of a number of texts, such as Bowe's *Handicapping America* (1978) and his *Rehabilitating America* (1980), Kleinfield's *The Hidden Minority* (1979), and De-Loach and Greer's *Adjustment to Severe Physical Disability: A Metamorphosis* (1981). According to the research summarized within these texts, voiced attitudes toward the disabled in the American society tend to be mildly positive, whereas unvoiced attitudes are often deeply hostile. Moreover, there is evidence that hostility toward those who depart from the social norm in a way perceived as undesirable is increasing (Lampos, 1981; Ramsey, 1978; Stein, 1978).

The early social movement aimed at creating a barrier-free environment reflected these attitudes. While the federal barrier-removal legislation of the late 1960s and early 1970s resulted from a voiced support of environmental accessibility, initially it produced no nationwide changes. Nevertheless, by the late 1960s some states and local municipalities had enacted accessibility codes that produced sporadic attempts to build ramps to buildings with steps, to install curb cuts at street corners with high curbs, and to install wide doors and railings in public restrooms. Several large motel chains, such as Holiday Inn and Travelodge, were pioneers in the attempt to provide accessible accommodations for disabled travelers.

In 1965 a report of the National Commission on Barriers to the Rehabilitation of the Handicapped identified architectural barriers and, especially, transportation barriers as the greatest social deterrents to the assimilation and employment of disabled people. The Commission's report resulted in the Architectural Barriers Act of 1968—the first federal legislation directed at eliminating the physical barriers that prevented access to buildings funded in whole or in part by the federal government. While enforcement of the Act was nonexistent in the years immediately following its passage, the establishment of the Architectural and Transportation Barriers Compliance Board (A&TBCB), through enactment of the 1973 Rehabilitation Act, resulted in explicit guidelines for reporting and dealing with violations of the 1968 Act. Transgressors were threatened by the withholding of government funds if they were found to be in violation of the law's intent.

By the mid-1970s, however, it had become apparent that problems existed concerning the Board's efficacy, largely due to the interests represented by many of the Board members. As Mace (1977) pointed out, "Ironically, the very make-up of the Board (members are heads of agencies such as the Department of Health, Education and Welfare, Department of Transportation, Department of Housing and Urban Development, Department of Labor, Department of the Interior, Department of Defense . . . ) has limited the effectiveness of the Board's compliance/enforcement efforts because each of the member agencies has construction activities and may be subject to compliance action which they can veto as members of the A&TBCB." According to Mace certain Board members actively worked to forestall the entire Board's attempts to enforce compliance and assist in the implementation of approved accessibility standards.

Eventually, however, the actions of the Board ended criticisms of its actions from one quarter, only to provoke criticisms from another. Before 1981 the approved accessibility standards were those of the American National Standards Institute (ANSI). In January of 1981, the A&TBCB completed its own revised set of accessibility guidelines, which set new minimum standards for facilities that federal agencies owned or leased. Six months after it completed the guidelines, the Board was severely censured for the exactness of the standards it had been mandated to develop and was threatened with extinction. Issuance of the improved standards created a furor "in several major newspapers and periodicals, as well as within the Reagan Administration" (Gorski, 1981). The Reagan administration responded to the Board's attempts to carry out its legislated task by recommending the Board not be funded for the 1981–82 fiscal year.

BARRIER-FREE TRANSPORTATION

Before establishment of the A&TBCB, the movement to eliminate barriers in public transportation and the movement to eliminate barriers in architecture were distinct. The Architectural Barriers Act made no specific mention of public transportation. In 1970 Congress attempted to rectify its oversight by passing the Biaggi Amendment to the Urban Mass Transportation Act of 1964. The

Biaggi Amendment established as federal policy that the disabled have the same rights to mass transportation services as other members of the public.

Congress continued to press for accessible transportation. Legislation first threatened to withhold the approval of the Secretary of Transportation from projects that did not allow for the access of disabled people to "public mass transportation facilities, equipment and services" (the 1974 Amendment to the 1973 Federal-Aid Highway Act) and finally threatened to withhold funds for the "purchase of passenger rail or subway cars . . . motor buses, or for the construction of related facilities unless . . . designed to meet the mass transportation needs of the elderly and handicapped" (the DOT Appropriations Act of 1975). In addition, regulations eventually issued in 1977 for Section 504 of the Rehabilitation Act of 1973 held that denying disabled people access to federally funded transportation services and facilities was in violation of their civil rights.

Attempts to implement existing legislation had barely begun when, in the summer of 1981, the Reagan administration eliminated the extension of the Rehabilitation Act of 1973, Section 504, to conveyances and facilities funded completely or in part by the federal government. Although maintaining that disabled people must still be provided with transportation services, the Reagan administration turned over to local municipalities the problem of how best to provide that transportation without financial support from the federal government. The controversy concerning accessible transportation services and the effect of inadequate services on the outcome of ILR efforts will be discussed in the concluding sections of this chapter.

## A BARRIER-FREE ENVIRONMENT AND LEVELS OF INDEPENDENCE

Without accessible architecture and transportation within their own communities, severely disabled people will be unable to attain their optimum levels of independent functioning. If barrier-free design is limited to settings in which disabled people receive medical services or in which they reside, then institutionalization and social isolation of such people will continue. The similarity between life in institutions designed to shelter and provide services to disabled persons and life in institutions established to punish or segregate public offenders has been noted by sociologists and rehabilitation professionals since the early part of this century (Lenihan, 1977). The major difference between institutions for the disabled and institutions for public offenders is that preferential treatment is more often given to those who violate social laws and regulations than to those who violate social standards of physical function and appearance. Unless deinstitutionalization of disabled people becomes an accepted social policy, people incarcerated because of committing a serious crime can expect to be paroled long before those who are incarcerated because of a physical or mental defect can expect to return to their communities, for the latter are often committed for life.

What opponents of the society-oriented philosophy of independent living (see Chapter 3) fear, however, is that without barrier-free communities to return to, disabled people may be discharged from mental hospitals and custodial care facilities to remain isolated within the general community. Without the necessary support services and without accessible community-wide environments, such people will continue to experience the restrictions of institutional living while being deprived of its benefits. If IL services are limited to increasing people's physical self-sufficiency in order to safely segregate them by themselves or with small groups of similarly disabled people, then independent living will no longer be a progressive social service philosophy.

In Chapter 2, the three levels of independent living were described in order to provide a framework for establishing and evaluating IL goals. We can now consider what environmental accommodations facilitate optimum function at each of these three levels.

INDEPENDENCE IN BED

A major IL goal for those who must spend most of their time in bed is barrier reduction within their immediate environment. This might consist in an uncomplicated device that allows a severely disabled person to use a telephone or in a more complex technological aid such as an environmental control system, which can permit a person who has voluntary control of only a few muscle fibers to adjust the position of the bed, moderate the temperature and lighting in a room, and activate or deactivate televisions, radios, tape-recorders, and voice synthesizers. Such environmental aids can bring the most severely disabled people to their highest level of independent functioning by permitting them to control their immediate environment and to communicate with other persons, either at a distance, through the telephone or teletypewriter, or face-to-face, through computer printouts or through computerized speech.

As at all other levels of independent functioning, safety is a primary concern for those who spend all or most of their time in bed. For people with this degree of impairment, a plan should be developed that would allow for a quick and convenient evacuation of the individual, the bed, and any necessary life support equipment in case of an emergency. In first floor bedrooms, sliding glass doors can be installed that are wide enough to allow a bed to pass through and that open directly to an outside ramped deck or ground level area. In addition to allowing for a rapid evacuation in an emergency, such a design also increases the chances for severely disabled people to have periodic excursions outside their homes.

At Timbers, a residential center for physically disabled young adults in Wichita, Kansas, the most severely disabled residents are housed in a single-storey building shaped like a huge triangle. Attached to the patio that extends from the base of the triangle is a wide, gently sloping ramp with 4-foot-high sides of solid concrete. This ramp leads from the community room to a large underground tornado shelter. Although Timbers accepts no residents with physical problems severe enough to confine them to bed, the safety features incorporated in its design could easily be adapted to the living situations of such people.

It should not be assumed, however, that people who must remain in their beds or who are dependent on life support systems cannot participate in activities outside their homes. In her book *Housing and Home Services for the Disabled* (1977), Laurie describes the efforts of disabled people in England to obtain services that would allow them to live at home, instead of in institutions. According to Laurie's description of the 1969 protest march that took place in the pouring rain in front of No. 10 Downing Street, "20 men and women in iron lungs on truck beds or using respirators in wheelchairs, led the parade" (1977, p. 7).

## INDEPENDENCE IN THE HOME

In the home barrier-free design is concerned with two major areas: architectural accessibility and assistive aids and devices.

**Barrier-Free Home Design**   In designing a barrier-free home, the basic elements of architectural accessibility must be considered: accessible entrances, usable storage facilities, counters, appliances, and bathroom fixtures of the correct style and installed at the appropriate height (see Chapter 10). Equally important, however, at this level of functioning are design factors that are often overlooked, such as the slope of the land on which a residence is situated and the texture of the surfaces over which a disabled person must move.

Wolfensberger (1978) points out that selecting a building site that does not allow a disabled person to move about the immediate outside area without assistance or complex mobility aids displays a lack of foresight. According to Wolfensberger, De Haupt, a Dutch residential center for disabled people, is an outstanding example of this kind of architectural blindness. Since De Haupt was built on an extremely hilly site, residents are forced to use motorized wheelchairs whenever they go outdoors. Such blunders are not unknown in the United States either. In Arlington, Tennessee, builders constructed hills on previously level ground, so that a developmental center for severely multiply handicapped children and adults could be constructed on top of steep slopes.

This unawareness of the importance of the natural physical environment to disabled people is reflected innumerable times in the building sites selected by families with disabled members. Emily E. has multiple sclerosis but is totally self-sufficient in her self-care and is able to do her housework from her wheelchair without assistance. But Emily's independence ends at her front door. The slope of the lot on which her home was built is so steep that she cannot wheel from her front door to the driveway without having someone with her who can keep her wheelchair from rolling into the street. Although the lot on which her otherwise accessible home was built was purchased after she could no longer walk, no one took into account the effect of the surrounding terrain on her ability to enter and leave her home without assistance.

Emily and her family did avoid the second most often overlooked accessibility feature in a home: inappropriate floor covering. For anyone who uses a wheelchair or walker, thick carpets can be a great impediment. For those who use canes or crutches, a greater hazard is posed by wet or waxed surfaces, or by area rugs that lie over smooth surfaces and that cause a cane or crutch to slip.

Design considerations in the home must take in not only a person's self-care and home-maintenance requirements, but also his or her avocational interests. Gas grills, installed at the appropriate height, permit people with hemiplegia or who use wheelchairs to cook outdoors safely without having ashes to dispose of. Similarly, raised indoor or outdoor planters installed at the most convenient height for someone in a sitting position, such as a quadriplegic, or someone who cannot bend down, such as a hemiplegic, can provide a home gardener with many relaxing hours.

A major problem faced by drafters of accessibility standards is that a design that eliminates barriers for people with one kind of physical limitation may create barriers for those with a different one. For example, a bathroom commode that is at a usable height for someone with advanced rheumatoid arthritis may be too high for someone with SCI quadriplegia. Whether one has lost the function in the left or right hand can also make a great difference in how well one can use refrigerators, washers, or dryers, or reach remote areas of cupboards when the door only opens in one direction. Many such mini-barriers, like the doors on refrigerators, can be eliminated by reversing the way the door is hung, but others may be more difficult to eradicate. When a commode seat is too high, the only solution may be to install another commode of the proper design. When a commode seat is too low, its height can easily be increased by commercially available seat heighteners. IL programs that have modular bathrooms in which clients can be evaluated and trained can help determine before a client's home is modified which particular adaptation best suits the client's strength, agility, and range of motion (May et al., 1974).

Because of the difficulty of drafting accessibility standards that accommodate the functional limitations of people with diverse disabilities, any standards used as a guide in modifying a home must be adapted to the specific individual's requirements. Even then, structural modifications alone will be unable to compensate for the functional limitations of severely disabled people. As Laurie (1977, p. 11) points out, "Adapting to a disability is a two-way street: the individual must adapt to the environment, and the environment must be adapted to the individual."

**Assistive Aids and Devices**  For most disabled people, the ability to function independently in the home depends on a variety of often inexpensive assistive aids and devices. An example is a category of devices of various designs called reachers. A reacher usually consists of a straight, either fixed or extensible, length of wood or metal with a pinching mechanism on one end and a controlling mechanism on the other. Reachers allow people who cannot raise or extend their arms or who have little strength in their fingers to lift objects on and off high surfaces, retrieve items from the floor, and, in the hands of a true adept, insert plugs into sockets and manipulate the controls on appliances.

Along with reachers, a wide range of inexpensive aids has been developed that can make the difference between needing assistance and independence in routine tasks. Among these are brailled control knobs for people with visual impairments and smoke alarms and doorbells that activate flashing lights to alert people with hearing impairments. A relatively recent innovation in this area is the use of trained animals to assist disabled people. While dogs have been used for decades by blind people, the use of dogs to supplement the communication skills of hearing-impaired persons is of more recent origin. Hearing-ear dogs, as they are called, respond to certain types of stimuli—such as fire alarms, kitchen timers, or telephones—by attracting their owners' attention and then leading him or her to the source of the sound. Both dogs and monkeys have been successfully trained to assist severely disabled people by bringing items to them on command and by picking up dropped items and placing them within their owner's reach. Monkeys have learned to feed high-level quadriplegics and eventually may be useful in assisting people with a wide range of disabling conditions.

Unfortunately, the use of animals to increase functional independence is not without drawbacks. While the user may become more independent through the use of well-trained animals, the animals will themselves be dependent in certain areas. Dogs and monkeys must be cared for, which can impose a new set of functional demands on severely disabled people. Nevertheless, although animals cannot substitute for a human attendant, they may reduce the need for assistance from other people in certain activities of daily living.

## INDEPENDENCE IN THE COMMUNITY

The oil shortage during the winter of 1973 and the following spring created economic reverberations that resulted in long-lasting alterations within American society. Transportation, both public and private, survived the immediate energy crisis only to face increased operating deficits and a future of steadily diminishing supplies of oil. Rising energy costs, with an accompanying high rate of inflation, threatened the existence of public transportation services in general. For severely disabled people, in particular, whose transportation needs were just beginning to be recognized, the implications were disasterous.

Eventually, the effect was felt by the network of support services essential to optimum ILR. Because independence within the community depends on severely disabled people being able to travel about the community, ILR could succeed in its entirety only if accessible modes of transportation were available.

**Privately Owned Modes of Accessible Transportation**   For those who can afford to purchase and operate them, modified cars and vans allow mobility within the community.

*Modified Cars*   Cars equipped with hand controls have been available since World War II. In order to use such cars independently, however, a person must be able to transfer in and out and to load and unload whatever mobility aid he or she uses, such as a walker or wheelchair. Although carlike vehicles have been designed that can be entered and driven from a wheelchair, they tend to be too expensive or too unreliable to provide a practical means of transportation for people who cannot transfer themselves in and out of standard cars.

Mass-produced automobiles that are brought off the assembly line and then modified pose several problems for a severely disabled driver. First, with the trend toward smaller, more energy-efficient vehicles, few cars have interiors large enough to allow a collapsed wheelchair or walker to fit behind the front seat. Second, many severely disabled people use motorized wheelchairs, which cannot be loaded into a standard car without being dismantled completely. Even the few models that have removable battery cases, power controls, and wheels are difficult to disassemble and reassemble without assistance. If the goal of accessible transportation is independent mobility, modified cars are not the answer for most severely disabled people.

*Modified Vans*   The number of disabled people who cannot use a modified car but could drive a modified van is unknown. Since the early 1970s, however, when wheelchair-accessible vans first became available to the general public, hundreds of companies specializing in van modifications have been established across the country. The proliferation of companies that modify vehicles for severely disabled drivers is more than matched by the number of different modifications.

For example, a modified van can have any one of a wide variety of side- or backloading wheelchair lifts and any of an equally wide variety of modified driving controls. Driving controls range from the simplest type of modification—where the driver uses one hand on a lever to accelerate and brake, while using the other to turn the steering wheel—to an extremely sophisticated type of control that cradles the forearm so that only minimal gross arm and shoulder movement is needed to accelerate, brake, and steer. As modifications increase in sophistication, they also increase in price. In 1979 a van with the simplest modification cost approximately $14,000, while one with the sophisticated modification described above cost $25,000. By 1980 a van with a driving control that cradled the forearm cost approximately $30,000. Fortunately, the increasing availability of used modified vans gives many people who could not afford a new vehicle the chance to own a modified van of their own.

One of the suggestions made by the Reagan administration to reduce the transportation problems of disabled people was that, in lieu of modifying mass-transit systems to make them accessible, the government should purchase a modified vehicle for everybody who needed one. If the Department of Transportation's estimate that there are 17.5 million people who cannot use unmodified public transportation is correct, the implications of this suggestion are staggering. To supply modified vehicles to just those people who acquire a severe disability from a spinal cord injury would be financially out of the question. Between 10,000 and 12,000 people, 75 percent of them between the ages of 16 and 26, become permanently disabled from spinal cord injuries each year. The most commonly acquired spinal injury is at the level of the fourth or fifth cervical vertebra, resulting in high-level quadriplegia (Hylbert and Hylbert, 1981), and high-level quadriplegics require the most sophisticated driving controls. If only 4,000 of the approximately 10,000 to 12,000 people injured each year required the cradle control described above, in one year, at 1980 prices, the cost of "suitably modified vehicles" would be approximately $116 million. This amount would not include the cost of replacing vehicles that were no longer operational or the cost of supplying private transportation to people with other severely disabling conditions.

## Public Modes of Accessible Transportation

*Taxi Service* For people with adequate incomes who can transfer with a minimum of assistance, taxis have long been the transportation service of choice. Unlike mass-transit systems, taxis provide door-to-door service, and drivers will often help passengers with bulky items. According to Goodkin (1977), 14 percent of the intracity travel of disabled people takes place in taxis; the figure for the general population is 2 percent.

Taxi service, unfortunately, is expensive, compared to other forms of transportation services. In 1973 the "Comprehensive Needs Study of Individuals with Most Severe Handicaps," conducted by the Urban League, revealed that 11 percent of severely disabled people were homebound because they could not get in and out of vehicles without assistance. Of those who could use taxis, the Urban League discovered, "25 percent spent

$11.00 a week and 6 percent over $76.00 a week" on transportation alone.

For those on fixed and limited incomes, using any transportation service that is operated for profit can be prohibitively expensive. But cost is not the only deterrent. As Goodkin (1977) points out, since most cabs no longer have a larger back seat, people who might otherwise have been able to transfer themselves in and out of the back of a taxi can no longer do so. Moreover, local laws often prevent any passengers, including disabled people, from riding in front alongside the driver. Finally, drivers may refuse to accept disabled people as passengers for a variety of reasons, the most common of which is their reluctance to lose the amount of time it takes for people with mobility impairments to get in and out of their cabs. Many people who use crutches, walkers, or wheelchairs have experienced the frustration of summoning a taxi, only to have it speed up and pull away when the driver realized that the would-be passenger was disabled.

*Private Van Services*   Minibus and private van companies that for a profit transport disabled people, including those who remain in wheelchairs, are available in many large communities. The primary function of these companies may be to provide emergency transportation services, but often they are the only means of transportation available to those who do not have modified vehicles of their own. In many communities, according to Goodkin (1977), private van services cost a minimum of $10.00 for a one-way trip with an increase in the base amount according to the distance traveled. Often, the cost of these services is prohibitive.

In Bal Harbour, Florida, in 1979 during the Wheelchair II Conference, a private van service was employed to transport disabled people to and from Miami airport at the cost of $75.00 per person for a one-way trip. The cost was established on a per person basis even though several people rode together in a single trip. As a result, the cost of transporting disabled participants to the Conference hotel and back to the airport exceeded the cost of flying them into and out of Miami airport. Clearly, while private van services provide a service that is valuable in emergencies, they do not provide a feasible solution to the day-to-day transportation needs of severely disabled people.

*Paratransit Services*   Paratransit describes any transportation services that provide vehicles which are designed to accommodate both ambulatory and wheelchair passengers and that are, usually, operated for profit. Paratransit services include "dial-a-ride, jitney, community mini-bus, subscription bus service, certain forms of van pooling and other types of collective transportation service" (*Urban Mass Transportation Act*, 1976). Paratransit does not include, according to the Urban Mass Transit Authority (UMTA), private cabs with no accessibility features.

For disabled people, the most successful kinds of paratransit services have been those operated as dial-a-ride systems directly by or through contracts with local public mass-transit systems. Initially, these dial-a-ride systems were intended to provide interim services until mainline mass-transit systems met the accessibility standards established under Secton 504. After transportation services for disabled people were taken out of the jurisdiction of Section 504 and became subject to the discretion of local mass-transit authorities, the dial-a-ride services, in most instances, moved from being an interim solution to being a permanent one. These dial-a-ride services have many of the advantages of taxi and private van services, in that they provide door-to-door services, and they have the additional advantage that most of the operating costs are met by government subsidies. In most areas, passengers on dial-a-ride systems pay the same fare as do people riding mainline bus systems.

Unfortunately, the advantages of low-cost, door-to-door dial-a-ride services are overshadowed by the fact that the need for such services far surpassed the estimates of national and local transit authorities. In August 1980 the Memphis transit authority subcontracted its dial-a-ride service, which was to operate seven accessible vans, to a local cab company that was quickly overwhelmed by the numbers of people eligible for and in need of services. At first, the priority system established by the Department of Transportation kept the system from chaos. First priority was given to trips to and from places of employment; second, to trips for educational purposes; third, to trips for medical purposes; fourth, to trips to meet basic living needs, such as grocery shopping; and fifth, to trips for personal business and pleasure. By December 1980, however, it was impossible to schedule a trip for any purpose from 7:00 to 10:30 in the mornings and from 3:00 to 6:00 in the evenings. At those hours, all available spaces were filled by people going to their jobs or classes. By August 1981 people with no reserved time slot were rarely able to schedule a trip at any time of the day or week.

The argument most often heard against making new mass-transit conveyances and systems accessible is that not enough disabled people need or could use barrier-free systems to render them worthwhile. That argument has been invalidated by the demand for existing barrier-free systems that are both affordable and reliable. Once the need had been established, however, a new argument was raised: the cost of incorporating accessibility features into newly built facilities, such as Amtrak stations, and newly purchased conveyances, such as trains, subway cars, and buses, was too costly to be acceptable.

*Modified Mainline Buses* Following the government's decision not to enforce legislation mandating barrier-free mass-transit systems, newspaper editorials across the country bore headlines like "Good Idea, Bad Policy" (*Daily Herald*, 30 July 1981, p. 4). The "good idea" was having either 50 percent of all mainline buses or 50 percent of the number of buses in operation during peak hours barrier-free by 1989. The "bad policy" was mandating the additional costs of accessibility features in new vehicles and facilities at a time when the federal government was seeking to reduce its role in funding public transportation in general. As the editorials indicated, there would be both advantages and disadvantages to a policy that would meet the transportation needs of disabled people by establishing accessible mainline transit services. The advantages would be the affordability to the customer and the cost-effectiveness over time. The disadvantages would be the inability of a certain percentage of people to use mainline systems and the high immediate costs of instituting such systems.

*Advantages* Unless paratransit systems are supported in part by public monies and keyed, therefore, to fares paid by users of local mass transit, their cost will far exceed the ability of most disabled persons to pay. Systems, like dial-a-ride, that are demand responsive, requiring time- and gas-consuming routing of vehicles, cannot be as cost-effective and reliable to operate as are fixed-route systems.

Because they are less expensive to operate, mainline bus services are more likely to survive reductions in operating budgets than are auxiliary services. In areas where transit funding has been reduced, dial-a-ride and paratransit systems were the first services to be abolished (Goodkin, 1977). Finally, in terms of cost-effectiveness over time, it has been estimated that the cost of making mainline buses wheelchair-accessible, whether by installing ramps, lifts, or floors that could be lowered hydraulically, if prorated over the estimated lifetime of a mass-transit bus "would average out to less than $1.00 per (disabled) person per year over the next 30 years" (Moakley and Weisman, 1981, p. 35), or cost on the average $95 per bus per year for the total disabled ridership (Lancaster, 1976).

*Disadvantages* Unfortunately, when the cost per transit conveyance, multiplied by the number of conveyances operating nationwide, is added to the cost of incorporating ramps and elevators in terminals and stations, the cost of totally accessible public transportation has been estimated to be from 2.5 billion to 6.8 billion dollars over the next 30 years (Jameson, 1981). Moreover, there is a question as to which type of transportation service will meet the needs of the largest proportion of disabled people. Paratransit systems provide the convenience of door-to-door service and drivers who can be specially trained to provide needed assistance to disabled people. A mainline system would mean that disabled people would have to be able to get to a bus or subway stop and to board and disembark without the assistance of the driver.

If accessible fixed-route systems ever become a reality, however, certain societal changes can be expected to occur that might enhance the efficacy of accessible mass transit. The question of how to provide the best service for the least money requires a careful analysis of those public transportation systems that are already accessible.

In 1981 the City of Chicago operated a paratransit system that provided "76,480 one-way trips for 1,583 persons" at a cost of $1,000,000. According to Moakley and Weisman (1981), Chicago's system was able to provide transportation to "less than 1% of Chicago's 281,700 handicapped persons because the system was unable to find any other way to keep ridership at a manageable level than to deny rides to the majority of persons who requested the service" (p. 23).

Much of the opposition to making mass transit barrier-free is based on estimates of how many disabled people use existing systems. According to Jameson (1981), "Of the 7,595 elevator riders at the 41 Washington, D.C., subway stations one day last April, the transit system reported, only 160 were in wheelchairs, blind or on crutches; the rest were able-bodied." One suspects, from the numbers Jameson cites, that more disabled people did not use the elevators because such people, especially those in wheelchairs, were unable to get into elevators that were crowded with people who were not disabled. Similarly, an article in *U.S. News and World Report*, 20 July 1981, entitled "Equal Access Not So Easy for Buses, Subways," states near the beginning of the article that, on the average, four people in wheelchairs ride the buses in Detroit each day. Further on, the article quotes the director of the Detroit Transportation Department, who states, "On a good day 20 percent of the lift-equipped buses aren't working. On a bad day, it's 40 percent" (p. 45). Apparently the author of "Equal Access . . . " did not perceive any relationship between low ridership and poorly designed lifts. What intelligent person would venture out into the community if the probability of becoming stranded was as great as it is for severely disabled people in Detroit?

As Moakley and Weisman (1981) point out, statistics on ridership of modified systems cannot give an accurate indication of the potential use of barrier-free systems for several reasons: first, unless the system is known to be reliable, the majority of potential users who are severely disabled will literally be unable to use the system; second, where reliable mainline systems do exist, feeder lines may remain inaccessible; and third, mainline systems may operate in communities that are largely inaccessible, so that curb cuts, reserved parking for disabled drivers, and accessible housing are not available. Each of these reasons can be eliminated. For example, reliable wheelchair lifts that are suitable for mass-transit systems are available and are in use in cities such as Seattle, where the proportion of disabled people using mass transit is high. Moreover, if federal, state, and local legislation that mandates barrier-removal is implemented, the communities in which mass-transit systems operate will eventually become accessible as curb cuts are installed and as public and privately owned buildings are constructed with ramps, elevators, and wheelchair-modified restrooms.

*Modified Rapid Transit Systems*   In terms of affordability and ease of use, barrier-free rapid transit systems are difficult to surpass, provided that disabled people can get to station terminals. The Washington, D.C., Metro, Atlanta's MARTA (Metropolitan Atlanta Rapid Transit Authority), and San Francisco's BART (Bay Area Rapid Transit) provide ease of access, low fares, and reliable transportation for people with severe mobility impairments.

The oldest of these three, BART, is the country's first accessible rapid transit system. At BART stations where the main entrance is below ground level, huge concrete ramps lead down to the entrance level, where elevators, available only to disabled people, provide rapid and protected access to the level from which the railcars depart. Once on the boarding level, people in wheelchairs can roll directly from the platform through wide, slowly closing doors into spacious railcars. BART cars ride so smoothly that, were it not for the possibility of a rail accident, it would not be necessary to lock the brakes on a wheelchair.

BART, unfortunately, lacks accessible feeder lines and has some stations with no parking places in the immediate area, so the number of disabled people who ride BART is not as high as it might otherwise be. Nevertheless, when the author departed Daly City on BART at 11:00 on a Wednesday morning, seven mobility-impaired people were leaving the station at the same time. The director of the Office of Handicapped Student Services at the University of California at Berkeley says that she, being in a wheelchair, finds it more convenient to ride BART than to drive herself into San Francisco on personal or University business.

*Long-Distance Travel: Airplanes and Trains* Accessible modes of long-distance travel are not as directly related to the day-to-day IL concerns of severely disabled people. Lack of barrier-free accommodations in long-distance travel affects only those who encounter job-related or recreation-related travel problems. Severely disabled businessmen and businesswomen must often drive long distances to business meetings or to conventions because of airline restrictions on carrying wet-cell wheelchair batteries. Inaccessibility in long-distance carriers also complicates the travel arrangements of IL programs that draw clients from a wide geographical area.

Most airlines, and the Amtrak system, have made some provisions for transporting disabled passengers, but these provisions mainly benefit less severely disabled people who can walk or use manual wheelchairs. In most large air terminals, airlines have personnel available who will assist disabled passengers with boarding and disembarking. If there are no boarding chutes available that allow people to enter planes directly from the terminal, passengers with severe mobility impairments are transferred into narrow boarding chairs, strapped in, carried up the boarding stairs, and then wheeled down the aisle to where their seat is located. Those who can transfer without assistance then do so, while those who need help are lifted into their seats by airline personnel.

At some small airports and with some airlines, severely disabled people may encounter certain difficulties with air travel. First, since different airlines have different policies, people with a severe mobility impairment are never certain, when they must transfer between planes on an indirect flight, whether or not they and their mobility aids will be allowed to continue on the second leg of the trip. Second, even within the same airline, different policies regarding the transportation of power wheelchairs may be in effect at different times. On one trip a person may not be allowed to fly with a motorized wheelchair. On a subsequent trip he may be told that he may take along his motorized wheelchair, but only if he uses a certain type of battery. Most airlines, if they will transport any wheelchair battery, will allow gel (semisolid conducting agent) batteries but will not allow batteries with wet cells (batteries filled with a liquid with a high acid content). On still another trip he may be informed that he can fly out with his motorized wheelchair and any type of battery he chooses, but on the return trip may be forced to leave the battery behind, leaving him completely immobile when he arrives back at his point of departure. Third, if a severely disabled person arrives at his destination and discovers that no accessible public transportation or paratransit services exist in the area, unless he can use a taxi or has friends nearby, he may be forced to remain at the airport until he can book a return flight.

Travel by train is often inconvenient for disabled people for two reasons: inaccessible Amtrak stations and an Amtrak policy that does not permit disabled people to remain in their wheelchairs while enroute. Very few Amtrak stations have platforms that are level with the floor of individual passenger cars, so in most stations mobility-impaired people cannot walk or roll directly from the platform into the railway car. Amtrak has, however, made certain provisions for disabled passengers, including designing rail cars with aisles wide enough to allow a wheelchair to pass. In addition, Amtrak policy calls for a minimum of one specially designed car on each train with accessible bathroom facilities. But while passengers were initially permitted to remain in their wheelchairs, recent policy changes require them to transfer into train seats and to have their wheelchairs removed to storage areas. Not only does this policy complicate train travel for the many people who are unable to transfer out of their wheelchairs without assistance, it also creates a problem when severely disabled people need to use the restroom facilities. First the wheelchair must be located and returned to them and then they must be lifted each time they need to go to the restroom or anywhere else.

## ROLE OF BARRIER-FREE ENVIRONMENTS IN INDEPENDENT LIVING

Clearly, the question of what transportation services should be available to disabled people has no easy answer. While the need for barrier-free transportation, like the need for barrier-free architecture, increases steadily with the growing percentage of disabled and elderly people in our society, the cost of barrier-free design is also increasing. The accessibility controversy is even more complicated than people who are not experienced in disability management might realize. Each type of specialized transportation service, like each type of architectural modification, will meet the needs of only a proportion of disabled people and, in certain instances, may actually inconvenience a different group of disabled people. For example, curb cuts on street corners can confuse blind persons who may walk onto the street without realizing they have left the sidewalk.

Nevertheless, barrier-removal efforts must be allowed to continue if disabled people are to become working members of American society. According to Goodkin (1977), 52.2 percent of disabled people between the ages of 17 and 64 are unemployed, and 67 percent of these could work "if accessible, low-cost transportation were available." The social cost of continuing to support the millions of unnecessarily unemployed disabled people who pay no taxes and who are on some type of income maintenance is not known, but estimates of that cost easily exceed the estimated cost of modifying all public transportation systems (Moakley and Weisman, 1981).

Goodkin estimates the minimum yearly cost of maintaining unemployed disabled people in terms of lost economic benefits— that is, unavailable goods and services, not counting lost tax revenues or increased welfare costs—at $824,000,000. If inflation is considered to affect cost of barrier-removal and cost of lost goods and services equally, modifying public transportation alone could result in an overall saving of 22.3 billion dollars over the next 30 years.

It is unlikely, because of factors of motivation or health, that all disabled people of working age would be willing or able to work. Moreover, continued high unemployment, coupled with continued prejudice toward disabled job seekers, makes it unlikely that the employment picture for disabled people will improve dramatically in the near future. Nevertheless, members of the House Education and Labor Committee, who testified in hearings on the proposed Gramm Latta II reductions in the vocational rehabilitation state grant program during the first federal budget debates in the summer of 1981, claimed that the 323,000 disabled people who would be unemployed without existing vocational rehabilitation (VR) services would cost "state, federal and local governments more than $196 million in lost taxes and increased public assistance in just one year" (*Word from Washington,* July 1981). The continued unemployment of just this relatively small proportion of disabled people, according to the congressmen, would cost the country $5.9 billion over a 30-year period. When seen as a choice between employment or continued joblessness, the $6.8 billion for accessible transportation over the same period seems less unreasonable than when it is given out of context.

Unfortunately, the relationship of a barrier-free environment to tax revenues, welfare costs, and the value of goods and services is not as clear-cut in analyses of the cost-effectiveness of ILR as of vocational rehabilitation. As explained in Chapter 4, it is difficult, if not impossible, to estimate the cost-effectiveness of ILR as a whole, much less any of the separate interdependent support services that are essential to ILR efforts.

One might argue that since employability is incidental to ILR, accessibility is less important in ILR than in vocational rehabilitation. But the reverse is true. The need for barrier-free transportation and architecture becomes apparent when one considers the role that an accessible environment plays in nonjob-related activities.

Every aspect of life in today's specialized, interdependent society depends to some degree on being mobile and, therefore, on having convenient access to innumerable business and leisure sites. If one imagines a world without wheels or without an energy source to operate those wheels, or a world where entrances to buildings—churches, homes, schools, banks—are high above the ground with no steps, ramps, ladders, elevators, or escalators to provide access, one sees more clearly the dimensions of the accessibility problem facing disabled people. Such a world demonstrates that the steps, stairs, and ladders of the nondisabled are the ramps, elevators, and escalators of the mobility-impaired. It illustrates that accessibility is a result of deliberate foresight and design. Architectural plans that allow for doors and steps can as easily allow for wide doors and ramped slopes to accommodate both those who walk and those who wheel from one place to another. Government surveys have shown that the cost of barrier-free design varies from no additional cost at all to one-tenth of one percent when accessibility features are incorporated into original building plans rather than added after construction has been completed. Modifying existing structures or existing transportation facilities and conveyances is significantly more expensive than accommodating the needs of disabled people from the outset.

If disabled people are to live at their optimum levels of independence, they must have more than the training and equipment that allows them to carry out their own self-care and home management routines. They must also be provided with a community-wide environment that permits them to go to the grocery store of their choice and select the foods they prefer, as well enabling them to prepare that food and clean up after their meals at home. They must be able to obtain the medical and dental care they require from the physician and dentist they prefer as well as being able to carry out prescribed health regimens at home. They must be able to meet with their friends and attend the religious services of their choice, instead of being relegated to passively waiting for someone to come to them to pass a friendly hour or deliver spiritual support. Too many times other people expect the disabled to be excluded from any active participation in community life. Even the term religious communities often use to describe their disabled parishioners—"shut-ins"—inaccurately describes these parishioners' true social situation, which is "shut-out." IL programs can open the door to more active, fulfilling lives, and barrier-free architecture and transportation are the two keys that unlock that door.

What can an IL program do to increase community accessibility or to make optimum use of what resources are already available? Depending on the resources a program has, the following goals could be incorporated into a service delivery plan:

1. Developing and maintaining a listing of accessible apartments, homes, and business places within the community.

2. Maintaining a resource library that has specific reference materials dealing with architectural accessibility, such as barrier-free kitchen and bathroom designs and copies of local, state, and federal accessibility standards and codes.

3. Establishing a reputation as a community resource in the area of accessibility, by offering information on standards and consulting with businesses and private individuals.

4. Conducting community education services that include among their objectives increasing public awareness of disabled people's environmental needs and keeping local businesses informed of any tax deductions for architectural modifications.

5. Surveying existing community agencies that provide transportation services to develop a registry of accessible vehicles in the community and to determine the eligibility requirements for utilizing any accessible transportation services.

6. Establishing a self-help network of disabled people who own and operate accessible vehicles, so that in emergencies one disabled person can provide transportation for another. (Clients who choose to participate in transportation self-help networks must be made aware of their personal liability if the person they are transporting is injured.)

7. Establishing a self-help network of people who live in accessible homes, in order to bring together those who do not want to live alone and those who need a place to live.

# 9

## Independence: The Goal of Multiple Human Services

A review of the case of a person currently involved in an ILR process reveals that he has been served by a private insurance company, a private home health agency, a private vocational rehabilitation counselor, a rehabilitation hospital, a state rehabilitation agency, a state department of human services, a public housing project, and an institution of higher education. Some of these agencies have rendered extensive services. Others have only been involved in minor assistance. The disabled individual has had to interact with a wide variety of professional human service workers in these various agencies.

Such is the nature of ILR. It requires the contributions of a large number of diverse human service agencies and professionals. Yet the continued use of misnomers, such as IL center, in this field implies that there is some centralized location or agency at which a person may be transformed from a dependent to an independent state. That is a narrow view of ILR that is soon abandoned by those who become involved in this complex service delivery system.

169

The number and diversity of the human service agencies that contribute to the ILR process constitutes a problem and a challenge for the professionals involved. Each worker needs to understand the overall ILR service delivery system, which is a problem since that system is quite complex. That problem is converted to a challenge when the worker realizes that an understanding of the overall service delivery system can contribute to his or her own effectiveness within that system.

The purposes of this chapter are

1. to present the ILR process in such a way that the reader can conceptualize the service delivery system necessary to make that process successful,

2. to present a graphic model of the ILR process that helps to explain the interaction of the client with the various agencies,

3. to describe briefly some of the categories of services necessary in the ILR process and the agencies responsible for delivering those services, and

4. to give examples that illustrate how various human service agencies and professionals come together to assist a disabled person to live more independently.

## INDEPENDENT LIVING REHABILITATION: A CONCEPTUALIZATION

In Chapter 1 it was said that the ILR process is owned by the disabled person. Rehabilitation, it was noted, is a process in which an individual is involved rather than something that is done to or for that individual. Yet it will be apparent by now that a large portion of this text is devoted to descriptions of the agencies and professional services that make independent living possible. These various agencies and services together constitute an ILR service delivery system. This delivery system is loosely organized and is sometimes ill-defined, and many people involved in it are so consumed by their own professional roles and activities that they are unaware of their contributions to it. For that reason the ILR service delivery system is vague in nature as well as recent in origin.

In an attempt to adequately conceptualize ILR it is important to include both process and service delivery system. The ILR process is similar to any rehabilitation process: in it a disabled person attempts to eliminate, reduce, or circumvent the barriers that prevent his or her effective functioning. In that process, as noted in Chapter 1, that individual may need the assistance of various professional workers and service agencies. The responsibility of the ILR service delivery system is to make that assistance available. The system includes medical rehabilitation, vocational rehabilitation, home services, residential care services, and a host of other services. When it works effectively, the disabled or elderly person has available the assistance he or she needs to complete successfully the ILR process. One of the primary objectives of IL service programs authorized by the "Rehabilitation, Comprehensive Services, and Developmental Disabilities" legislation of 1978 is to ensure that the service delivery system does indeed function effectively.

## INDEPENDENT LIVING REHABILITATION: A NARROW VIEW

The ILR programs authorized by the 1978 Rehabilitation Amendments represent an attempt by Congress and the rehabilitation community to make IL services generally available to those who need them. When discussing IL services, many rehabilitation professionals have in mind the services authorized by that legislation. These service programs have both a very narrow and a very broad role in the overall ILR service delivery system.

The narrow role of these programs is that of direct service provider. The vocational rehabilitation agency of each state or, in some cases, some other appropriate public or private, nonprofit organization, may apply for grants of federal money in order to implement IL service programs. These grant funds can be used to rent office space, hire staff, pay for utilities and supplies, and meet other administrative needs. In addition, they may be used to provide direct services, such as attendant care and assistance with housing and transportation. So far, the amounts of money actually appropriated for these programs by Congress have been relatively small. Some states, for example, have received grants of only $200,000 to implement services for an entire state. Since overhead and other administrative costs must be paid first from these funds, the amount of money remaining for direct client services is reduced even further. The state/federal IL service programs, therefore, are not able to provide many direct services.

It should be noted that even though direct service provision is limited in these programs it is still an important function. Some of the services provided by these programs are critically important and not available from any other source.

Thus, direct service provision is an important but limited aspect of the state/federal IL programs. Similarly, it would be incorrect to view the state/federal programs as the primary component of the ILR service delivery system. These programs have a much broader role to fill in a much broader service delivery system.

## INDEPENDENT LIVING REHABILITATION: A BROADER VIEW

It has already been mentioned that the ILR service delivery system is a loosely organized collection of human service agencies and professional workers. Some of these agencies are clearly related to the objectives of ILR, such as Social Security and Medicare assistance. Others, such as public transportation and public housing programs, help to meet important IL needs even though that is not their primary objective. The state/federal IL service program is unique among these agencies in that its single purpose and objective is to enhance its clients' ability to live independently. To envision the ILR service delivery system in the broadest and clearest way, one should see the state/federal programs as filling a broad, coordinating role directing the attention of many diverse human service agencies to the needs of those involved in the ILR process.

It is important that the professional staff members of the state/federal IL service programs assume this coordinating responsibility. Even though most of the services that assist a person to live independently have been available in the past, there has not been a concerted, successful IL service effort because that key professional who would assume overall case management responsibility has not existed. That gap is now being filled by IL services staff members.

## INDEPENDENT LIVING: PROCESS AND SERVICES

As noted in Chapter 1, the disabled or elderly person plays the central role in ILR. The staff members of the state/federal IL service programs also play key roles, and a number of other agencies and professionals have necessary functions as well. This section will outline the way in which the client and an individual agency interact in the ILR process. (Since this outline focuses on client movement through the process, it is applicable to any agency involved in providing IL services.) The discussion will then be expanded to describe the various services and service agencies that may become involved in the process.

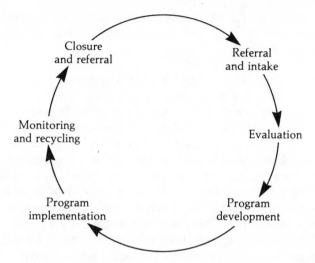

*Figure 9.1    Model of the independent living rehabilitation process.*

## PROCESS

Figure 9.1 represents the ILR process. The process has six stages, and it is portrayed as a circle to suggest that the client moving through it is involved in a series of cycles in which, with the help of successive IL agencies, he or she progressively moves toward greater independence.

**Stage One: Referral and Intake**    The first step is to involve the person who needs IL services. The referral and intake functions of any agency are sometimes overlooked or taken for granted, but they are important responsibilities. Almost all public agencies have the responsibility to make their services known to their communities so that people needing them will be made aware of their availability. Private agencies also seek referrals from their communities, in order to ensure that they have a sizable client population. One should note here that the primary responsibility of ensuring that potential clients are aware of services belongs to the service providers rather than to the clients.

Educating the community is not enough by itself to make the referral and intake stage successful. Each agency must also establish regular procedures by which it will receive referrals, make referrals to other agencies, and ensure effective two-way communication between referring agencies. McGowan and Porter (1967), Bitter (1979), and G. N. Wright (1980) all list important referral guidelines. A common theme from all sources is that referrals should be received and processed promptly, and that referral sources should receive feedback regarding the results of their referral.

**Stage Two: Evaluation** After getting a potential client into the process, the next thing that must be done is to identify the client's needs. This is referred to as evaluation or as needs assessment. In many agencies this stage will begin in the initial contact with the client, when he will be asked to state his needs as he perceives them. In some agencies a large amount of information will be collected from and about the client through a variety of highly technical procedures. This is true of medical rehabilitation centers, in which evaluation will probably involve extensive medical diagnostic procedures. Some agencies might ask the client to take a variety of psychological tests or to perform certain physical tasks under standardized conditions, in order to acquire carefully measured information. Finally, some agencies will seek to establish baseline data regarding the client's proficiency in certain skills essential to IL.

Depending upon the specific agency, any one or all of the above evaluation techniques may be used with clients. All agencies, however, have common objectives. The evaluation process should result in the identification and documentation of the client's functional limitations. Furthermore, all barriers, both internal and external, that lessen the client's ability to live independently should be identified. In practical terms this stage results in a clear statement of client problems, skill deficiencies, external barriers, and functional limitations.

**Stage Three: Program Development** Once the client's needs and problems are clearly identified, the client and the professional worker together can decide upon feasible and desirable goals and develop an action program to achieve those goals. Often the process of setting goals is as simple as turning each problem or skill deficit into a goal. For example, if the client is unable to dress independently then his or her goal would be to acquire the ability to do so. In other cases, the physical or mental restrictions of the client must be considered in setting goals. For example, some clients with severe physical restrictions may have to decide exactly what level of independence in personal care they think is desirable and attainable and then set that level as their goal.

Goal setting is the first step in the program development stage, but to achieve goals carefully designed action plans are necessary. The client and the professional worker must identify each step that the client needs to take to move from where he is to where he wants to be. This action plan should identify all available resources that might assist the client and should specify how and when these resources will be used. If outside services or people will participate, then the plan should specify what they will do and when they will do it. The plan should also specify when and how the program will be monitored and who will be responsible for that.

**Stage Four: Program Implementation**  The fourth stage is the simplest to describe. Here the program should be implemented as previously planned. It is important that the client, the professional worker, and any others involved follow the planned action steps carefully. If the plan is not carefully followed, then the later monitoring stage should catch that error.

**Stage Five: Monitoring and Recycling**  It is vital that the action program be monitored carefully. It is a good idea to have it monitored by both the client and the professional worker. They should have regularly scheduled times at which they evaluate the effectiveness of the program and progress toward the program goals. In addition, they should be constantly alert for early signs of anything going awry.

Specifically, they should monitor the client's progress in the IL skills specified as goals. If the client is achieving gains in those skills as anticipated, then no corrective action is necessary. If, however, the client is not progressing at the anticipated rate, then the client and worker should be prepared to reevaluate their action plan and take whatever corrective actions are necessary. In some cases the reevaluation may indicate that the action steps are appropriate but that the goals themselves are not. Perhaps more time is needed for goal achievement, or perhaps the client will decide, after some experience in the program, to change his or her goals slightly. While one should not simply change the goals of a program to fit what the person has actually achieved, and thereby lose all sense of challenge, success, or failure, one should be able to recognize when the goals specified originally are inappropriate and need to be changed.

In some cases the worker and client may not be able to determine why an action plan is not achieving the desired results. To identify the problem in such cases, it is helpful to retrace the steps of the entire process. First, check to see if each action step has been taken as planned. Incomplete or ineffective actions could be the problem. If that does not reveal the problem, then reexamine closely the entire action plan. A poorly drawn map will not lead one to the intended destination, and neither will a poorly designed action plan. If the problem is still not found, instead of becoming frustrated and feeling hopeless, as many do, return to the evaluation stage. It is likely that client needs, functional limitations, skill deficits, and external barriers have not been correctly identified. In that case the action plan was based on faulty data and has hardly any chance for success.

There is one other issue to be raised in the monitoring stage. What if the plan appears to be working? Do not automatically assume that no action is necessary. If the client is achieving the goals specified in the action plan, he may be feeling encouraged to raise those goals and strive for still greater independence. If that is the case, the client should be recycled. That is, the client and the worker should go back to the evaluation stage, establish a new baseline of skill levels, develop new goals, a new program, and begin implementing and monitoring that program.

**Stage Six: Closure and Referral**   The final stage of the ILR process cycle is closure and referral. This stage is identified in this way to indicate that the fact that one agency's contribution to the client is complete does not mean that he or she is finished with the process. Instead it probably means that the client is ready to move on to a different cycle.

To determine when a particular agency should close and refer an IL case, one should look at goal attainment. The client may have achieved all stated goals in his or her action plan and be satisfied that there are no further gains to be made with this IL service agency. For example, the client may have achieved all the physical recovery he or she currently believes to be possible in a medical rehabilitation center, and be ready to leave that center to participate in a community-based IL program that will provide additional training and services in the client's home.

In other cases it may become apparent that a client cannot achieve any further gains in a particular program even though such gains would be highly desirable. In those cases, a referral might be made to a program that offers more intensive treatment and services. For example, a client trying unsuccessfully to participate in a community-based program may decide that he or she needs further physical therapy and other medical rehabilitation services in order to acquire the skills needed for success in the community-based program.

In either of these cases, the agency's final disposition of the case is to make an appropriate referral. The reader may already be asking: Is the client ever finished with this ILR process? Does not this mean that the client is always a client and is never independent? As mentioned in earlier chapters, severely disabled and elderly people do sometimes achieve independence for very long periods. It has also been noted, however, that IL services of various kinds may be needed from time to time to help him or her to maintain that independence. G. N. Wright (1980, pp. 733–734) states that IL services can be used to prevent dependency, to rehabilitate for independence, or to maintain independence. It is to ensure that independence is maintained that referral is listed as the final disposition of any case. The client needs to know where he or she should go for services if needs arise in the future.

## SERVICES

The previous section has portrayed a process model through which the ILR client moves, usually with the assistance of some service agency. The number of such agencies can be quite large. Goldenson et al. (1978) list federal programs that provide assistance to disabled people. The list is over six pages long. Their list of voluntary organizations is some fifteen pages in length. Many of these voluntary organizations are important direct service providers.

Because of the very diverse range of services pertinent to IL and the large number of service providers, authors have had to categorize services in order to discuss the more prominent service agencies. DeLoach and Greer (1981), for example, classify services as self-care, educational, vocational, transportation, and residential. G. N. Wright (1980) discusses IL services under the headings of activities of daily living, adaptive devices, support services, housing, accessibility, and recreation. In the following discussion, case studies serve to illustrate the common services and agencies.

The reader should note that this is not an attempt to list all possible services and to describe all service agencies. The services needed by disabled and elderly people are as numerous and as individual as the people themselves, and the list of all service providers is not only long but constantly changing. To obtain specific information about the services available in a particular area, one should contact the local chamber of commerce or public library. Most communities have directories of all human service agencies in their area, and these directories are usually available in the public library. Sometimes bound copies are available for purchase from the chamber of commerce, library, or some other source. These directories are usually updated periodically and are the best source of current information.

## CASE ONE: ELEANOR M.

Eleanor was introduced in Chapter 2 as an 84-year-old widow who lives alone, had a total hip replacement, spent some time in a nursing home, and after a second hospitalization was able to return home.

First, note that Eleanor has been through at least two cycles of the ILR process. The first cycle was medical in nature. In it Eleanor's physician evaluated her needs and found that she was being limited by a diseased hip. A plan of action was developed (that is, surgery) to remedy that problem as much as possible. After that plan was executed, Eleanor's progress was monitored, and it was determined that she would need to continue her treatment in a nursing home. Later, after continued monitoring and further problems, Eleanor decided to arrange for an alternative course of action on her own. At that point she began a second cycle of the ILR process. She evaluated what she would need to live at home instead of in the nursing home. She served as her own case manager in developing a plan of action based upon her goal of living at home and her knowledge of her functional limitations. She proceeded to implement that plan of action, monitored its effectiveness, made changes in it that led to an even greater level of independence (she was able to dispense with the nurse's visits), and is continuing to live by herself. Eleanor may soon be at the point where she will begin still another cycle, since she is currently experiencing pain in her right hip and knee.

To effectively complete this ILR process, Eleanor has needed specific support services. The services and service agencies involved are described below.

*Medical* Obviously Eleanor has been served by a competent physician, physical therapist, nursing staff, hospital, nursing home, and public health nurse. The public health nurse visits were provided by the county health department at no cost to Eleanor. All the other medical services were provided at their usual cost. Most of these expenses were paid by Medicare, for which Eleanor is eligible since she is over 65 years old and is receiving Social Security benefits. Eleanor was fortunate in also having a private insurance policy to supplement Medicare, and, as a result, her medical fees were fully covered.

*Home Services* The first requirement for Eleanor to be able to live at home is an adequate income. Again Eleanor is fortunate in that she receives Social Security retirement benefits, and she receives some money from her late husband's retirement program and insurance policy.

After she returned home, Eleanor received one hot meal each day through the Committee on Aging, which is a local organization funded in part by the Comprehensive Older Americans Act Amendments of 1978. That program also offers counseling and advocacy services, assistance in locating appropriate housing, and recreational services to elderly people.

Some very important services were provided to Eleanor at no cost by volunteers who are active in a local senior citizen's group and in the Committee on Aging. These volunteers helped Eleanor with her housework, shopping, and other miscellaneous chores until she was able to do those things herself.

## CASE TWO: SUSAN J.

Susan is eight years old and is multiply handicapped. She attends a special school for severely disabled children. She can feed herself, but she is totally dependent for personal care upon her parents. As mentioned in Chapter 2, the primary concern of Susan's parents is to find some place that will take care of their daughter after they are no longer able to do so. Several areas of service are important for Susan.

*Financial Aid* Susan's parents, like most parents, were not prepared financially for the birth of a severely disabled child. Both her parents had worked full time before Susan was born, and they had expected that Susan's mother would be able to return to fulltime work within a few months after childbirth. They could not find a suitable child-care facility, however, and Susan's mother did not return to work after the birth. She has begun to work again in a parttime position now that Susan is in a public school. Her job enables her to be at home when Susan leaves for and arrives from school. She has not yet decided if she will be able to keep this job through the summer months, however, because of Susan's child-care needs.

Susan's parents have adjusted to having only one income, but there are still a number of financial troubles. Since Susan's father earns enough to put the family above established economic cutoff points, Susan is not eligible for Supplemental Security Income or for Medicaid. As a result the family depends on the group insurance policy from the father's job to pay Susan's medical bills. That policy covers most of these bills, but the family still has to budget for greater than average medical expenses.

Their financial situation has had an influence on a number of other important family issues. Susan's parents decided to postpone having any additional children until they had some feasible arrangements worked out for Susan. Now they are beginning to think that they will be too old for more children even if they do place Susan in a residential facility.

*Adaptive Devices* As mentioned in Chapter 2, Susan has a number of adaptive devices, which have been supplied for her through the assistance of a rehabilitation engineering center. Her father's group insurance policy covered most of the cost of these devices under its major medical benefits.

*Educational and Residential Services* As a result of the Education of All Handicapped Children Act of 1975, the public school system offers a special program for severely disabled children. Susan's teacher is attempting to help her learn basic self-help skills such as grooming and personal care. Susan is seen each week by a physical therapist, who leaves instructions for exercises that her teacher helps her to do each day. Susan's teacher and parents talk regularly about her educational program. Their cooperative efforts are helping Susan to make progress in some areas, and, equally important, they are preventing any deterioration in others.

Susan is involved in her current high-quality educational program as a result of her living at home. If she were in an institution she would not participate in the local school system's educational program, but would instead be provided with similar services within the institution. Susan's parents believe that her living at home and attending the local school system more effectively meets her needs than would an institution. This is another factor that makes it difficult for them to decide what options are best for Susan both now and in the future.

*Other Services* Susan and her parents are receiving services from several sources already. Yet there is a gap in the available services that could be very important to them. A small community-based group home for more severely disabled individuals could offer Susan the home atmosphere and community-based support services that seem to work for her quite effectively. Yet even though the number of group homes and other community-based alternatives to institutions is growing, there is very little to offer the more severely involved client. Recent texts by Laurie (1977) and by Flynn and Nitsch (1980) indicate that there is a great need in this area, but very few programs available to meet it. If such a program existed, Susan could continue to stay at home with her parents until such times as it was in her and their best interest for her to move into the group home. Then her move would be little different from that of any child growing up and moving away from her parents for the first time.

One other service, not now available in many places, that could be invaluable to Susan's parents is a respite care service. Occasionally Susan's parents need to travel out of town on family business. Having a respite service available that would provide competent attendant care for Susan while they were gone would make those trips much less demanding. They could also enjoy a short vacation periodically without taking Susan along. Respite care services have been implemented by nonprofit volunteer organizations in some communities, but unfortunately they are not available to Susan and her parents.

## CASE THREE: ERNIE C.

Ernie also was introduced in Chapter 2. He is a 19-year-old quadriplegic. He is independent in dressing, grooming, and personal care, and he can drive his own car with hand controls. Ernie has made no effort, however, to learn a vocational skill, or to learn the homemaking and cooking skills that he would need to live by himself. Instead he has continued to live at home, where he is dependent upon his parents in those areas. Recently Ernie met Ruth, and his relationship with her has caused him to want to find a job and move into his own apartment.

So far Ernie has been through a medical rehabilitation process, and he has learned the skills necessary for personal independence. Now he is ready and eager to move on to living on his own. The services Ernie has received and will receive in his ILR process are outlined below.

*Medical* Ernie is covered by a private insurance policy, which has paid almost all the medical expenses he has incurred. That insurance coverage is from his father's group policy at his job. Ernie is not eligible for Medicare, since he is not a Social Security recipient. He is not eligible for Medicaid either, but since eligibility for Medicaid is determined largely by financial need, he might become eligible if he moves away from home and is no longer dependent upon his parents.

Ernie's medical expenses have not been a problem so far, but he will need to plan carefully for them in the future. If he establishes his independence from his parents, then his father's group insurance will no longer cover him, and at that point he will need to have some other medical insurance coverage arranged. Hopefully, that coverage will come with a group policy at his own job.

*Home Management Skills*   As Ernie has begun to search for assistance in finding his own apartment and in learning the skills necessary to live alone he has been referred by a friend to a local IL center. This center is funded by the state/federal rehabilitation program. The staff of the center have met with Ernie and have developed with him a comprehensive program of services.

The staff and Ernie have planned for him to proceed with learning homemaking and cooking while he is in the process of finding and arranging to live in his own apartment. An occupational therapist who works parttime for the center has evaluated Ernie's physical abilities and has begun teaching him how to make his bed, vacuum floors, cook, wash dishes, and so on. The occupational therapist has visited Ernie's home, has surveyed its kitchen, and has talked with Ernie's parents. Ernie can begin practicing most of his homemaking skills in his parents' home, but their kitchen is only of limited usefulness to him because of its inaccessibility. The oven is built into the wall at a height that Ernie cannot reach and the range controls are behind the burners instead of in the front where Ernie could safely reach them. Because of these and other problems, Ernie will be practicing his cooking skills in a kitchen at the IL center. Ruth has also offered to let Ernie practice his cooking in her apartment, whose kitchen is more accessible than the one in his home.

*Social and Sexual Skills*   The second major activity in which Ernie has become involved at the IL center is a group counseling program. This group of staff members and clients meets once each week to discuss a wide variety of social and personal concerns. The group members help to support each other's attempts to become fully integrated into their communities. The issue that most concerns Ernie—and some of the other group members as well—is sex. His relationship with Ruth is causing him to wonder about how his disability might affect others' response to him as a sexual being. He also wonders if his physical limitations preclude any sexual activity. In the group counseling sessions, Ernie is learning that many other disabled people are enjoying healthy sex lives, and he is beginning to see that his sexuality is not affected by his disability as much as he had feared. In one special group session, several of the group members came with their wives, husbands, boyfriends, or girlfriends. Some couples attended in which one partner or both had been disabled for several years. In that session sexual activity and sexuality in a broader sense were discussed frankly and openly. Ernie and Ruth attended the session, and they were able to begin a healthy dialogue about this subject, which they had both been avoiding.

*Educational and Vocational Services*   The most certain route to full independence in this society is to have a job and to earn one's own living. In order to get a job that can meet his present and future needs, Ernie must acquire a marketable skill. For help in this area, the IL center staff referred Ernie to the state vocational rehabilitation service. The vocational rehabilitation counselor arranged for a comprehensive vocational evaluation program in which Ernie explored the many careers available to him and was tested to determine his vocational skills, aptitudes, and interests. As a result of the evaluation, Ernie decided to prepare himself for a career in business management, which means that he will need to enroll in college. His vocational rehabilitation counselor is assisting him to arrange to attend a nearby university that offers special services to its disabled students. Ernie's parents are willing and able to pay for his basic tuition and books, and the vocational rehabilitation agency has agreed to pay a maintenance fee that Ernie can use to offset his additional living expenses at the university. Since Ernie and Ruth are thinking about getting married, he hopes to find an accessible apartment near the campus where they can continue to live after their marriage.

## CASE FOUR: MARIE S.

Marie, who is mentally retarded, has lived in an institution for the past 43 years. All services have been provided in the institution. It has been home, hospital, school, and community for her. As a result of her long tenure in the institution, she is afraid to move out into a community-based group home.

If Marie ever moves into the group home, she will likely receive a variety of services. The home itself is funded by the state department of mental retardation. Marie's room and board in the home would be subsidized by Supplemental Security Income and Medicaid. In the community Marie might be involved in a sheltered workshop, in which she could earn an amount of money determined by her productivity. The workshop is operated by a local nonprofit corporation, and it is funded in part by the state mental retardation and vocational rehabilitation agencies.

Before Marie would be ready to move to a community-based group home she would need a great deal of preparatory training in the institution. First, because of her fear, she would need an adjustment program designed to enable her to leave the institution for short periods. The excursions could be increased slowly in frequency and in length to allow her to explore the outside

TABLE 9.1  CLIENTS, SERVICES, AND SERVICE PROVIDERS

| Client | Services | Service provider | Fees paid by: |
|---|---|---|---|
| Eleanor M. | Medical care | Physician | Medicare and insurance |
| | | Hospital | Medicare and insurance |
| | | Physical therapist | Medicare and insurance |
| | | Nursing home | Medicare and insurance |
| | | Public health nurse | No fee to Eleanor |
| | Financial support | Social Security | Social Security Administration |
| | | Private retirement funds | Private investments |
| | Meals at home | Committee on Aging | Committee on Aging |
| | Shopping and home chores | Volunteers | None |
| | Counseling, housing assistance, recreation (not used by Eleanor) | Committee on Aging | Committee on Aging |
| Susan J. | Financial support | Parents—Susan not eligible for SSI | Parents |
| | Medical | Personal insurance | Personal insurance |
| | Adaptive aids | Rehabilitation Engineering Center | Personal insurance |
| | Education | Public schools | Public schools |
| | Physical therapy | Public schools | Public schools |

| | | |
|---|---|---|
| Group home (not used by Susan) | Department of Mental Retardation | Department of Mental Retardation |
| Respite care (not used by Susan) | Local nonprofit volunteer organization | Local nonprofit volunteer organization |
| Ernie C. | | |
| Medical | Local hospital Rehabilitation hospital | Personal insurance Personal insurance |
| Home management services | Independent living center | Independent living center |
| Social and sexual counseling | Independent living center | Independent living center |
| Vocational guidance | State vocational rehabilitation agency | State vocational rehabilitation agency |
| Education and training | Public university | Parents and vocational rehabilitation agency |
| Marie S. | | |
| Residential | Institution Group home (not used by Marie) | Department of Mental Retardation SSI/Medicaid |
| Sheltered work (not used by Marie) | Local nonprofit corporation | Department of Mental Retardation Vocational rehabilitation agency Corporate income |
| Community living preparation (not used by Marie) | Institution | Department of Mental Retardation Volunteers |

world. At the same time as she is learning to cope emotionally with leaving the institution, Marie would need to be involved in a training program designed to teach her the homemaking and social skills necessary for success in the group home. These services would, of course, have to be provided by the institution, although volunteer workers would help Marie explore the outside world.

In the four cases just described, 14 broad categories of services were mentioned. Five of those categories of services were rendered to two or more of the clients. The other nine categories were unique to one case. Services were provided or paid for in these cases by over two dozen different service providers. Table 9.1 provides a summary of the clients served, services provided, and service providers.

The service providers listed in Table 9-1 make up a major part of the ILR service delivery system. When directed to the needs of a disabled or elderly person they can greatly facilitate that person's movement through the ILR process.

## SUMMARY

The intention of this chapter has been to demonstrate that an effective IL process is the result of a coordinated effort from a wide variety of human service agencies. A conceptualization has been offered for both the ILR process and the ILR service delivery system. Several case examples were used to illustrate how an individual involved in the ILR process interacts with and utilizes the services of the agencies and professionals who make up the service delivery system. It was suggested that an important, emerging role of the recently established state/federal IL service programs is to assume responsibility for case management in order to ensure that the appropriate service providers are involved in each individual's IL program at the appropriate time.

# PART THREE

*Varying Prototypes for
Independent Living*

# 10

## The American Dream:
## A Home of One's Own

One of the most vigorously defended rights in American society is the right to choose the location and conditions of one's own residence. This is especially true of elderly people, as indicated by the fact that 87.5 percent of all Americans over 65 years of age live in their own homes, with only 8.5 percent living in relatives' households and 4 percent in institutions (Brotman, 1976; Palmore, 1972). Research in Great Britain (Brearly, 1977) indicates a similar attitude, with only those elderly who cannot care for themselves, or who have no adequate accommodations, filing applications for residential care facilities. Although exact statistics for disabled people are not available, experience indicates that a similar attitude prevails. In the United States, the very establishment by disabled people of increasing numbers of independent living centers is evidence of the priority given to residential independence. So is the fact that many of these centers offer only training in independent living skills or support services to help people maintain their current level of residential independence and do not offer facilities for long-term occupancy. Other recent trends

**189**

indicating the desire of disabled people for residential independence are the rising number of apartment builders who include some accessible units in their new construction and the availability of specially designed manufactured housing to meet the needs of those with various mobility impairments. Both of these trends will be discussed in later sections of this chapter.

This chapter is organized around the three major types of independent housing available: private homes, manufactured housing (mobile homes), and apartments. Although these types of housing vary widely in size, cost, style, and other characteristics, they all offer options to the resident significantly different from those of less independent alternatives such as group homes or institutions. The advantages and disadvantages of each type of housing for the elderly or disabled person will be discussed, with specific suggestions for possible modifications for more convenient living. Sources of further information and some current cost estimates will be included.

## PRIVATE HOME OWNERSHIP

As in most areas related to housing, statistics are not available on the number of disabled people who now own their own home. It is known that about two-thirds of those over age 65 do own the home they live in, although these homes are often located in less desirable areas of town, so that their property value is less than average. The disabled person's reasons for wanting to own a home are similar to those of the nondisabled. Residential independence provides a sense of dignity, freedom, and stability, especially to elderly and disabled people (Maguire, 1979). Owning a home is seen as security against being placed in an institution against one's will. The comfort and familiarity of one's own neighborhood are reassuring and promote a sense of safety. Maguire (1979) indicates that older people who are moved out of their homes and neighborhoods often become disoriented in their new surroundings, and this contributes to both depression and accidents.

### ADVANTAGES

Ownership of one's own home is the ideal of most elderly and disabled people, and justifiably so in many respects. It not only provides security and freedom but also has other important benefits. One does not have to obtain permission to make any modifications to the exterior or interior of the home, and changes can be as permanent as desired. Huttman (1977) found that environmental control, such as decorating, having a personal garden, choosing one's furnishings, and having private living and storage areas, was very important to happiness. Especially with elderly people, the preference for familiar decorations and furniture inside the home extends to the neighborhood outside. Adjustment to new surroundings and new neighbors is more difficult for them because, in addition to the recognized deterioration in reaction time, sensory acuity, and other physical functions, elderly people have less stress tolerance than younger people (Huttman, 1977). The accumulation of equity in a long-term residence has the advantage of relieving some stress, since it is a form of financial insurance.

## DISADVANTAGES

Huttman (1977) notes that about 25 percent of those over age 65 are generally considered to be poor, yet Leeds (1973) states that the average elderly couple spend 34 percent of their income on housing, rather than the 25 percent usually recommended. This financial situation has certainly not been improved by the ever-increasing rates of inflation and property taxes, since the periodic government adjustments of retirement and disability incomes never keep up with rising costs. Even though elderly people usually have fewer physical, financial, and social resources than the average person—and this is often true of disabled people too—they are reluctant to give up a longtime home. In the case of disabled people, home ownership is frequently seen as central to a mainstream lifestyle, and anything else is seen as less desirable. Both elderly and disabled people, however, often have a reduced ability to do independently all the maintenance, cooking, cleaning, and other chores associated with home ownership (Huttman, 1977). Specific problems, as well as solutions, related to modifications and comfort and safety will be discussed in other sections of this chapter.

## OPTIONS

If the person is determined to move into, or remain in, a house in spite of the obstacles mentioned, there are some changes that may make the choice more financially and psychologically pleasant. Leeds (1973) found that the average elderly household had three rooms per person, or more than twice the space of younger poor families. This suggests the possibility of either converting the house into a duplex or renting out some rooms, perhaps with a private entrance. The same alternatives would apply to prospective disabled homeowners, with the addition that if attendant care is needed on a limited basis, the renter could be given a reduced rate for providing certain specified services such as cooking, laundry, or transportation. If one rented to a nonattendant, the rental income could pay for the hiring of someone else to provide the needed services. When careful screening is done prior to renting, a trustworthy renter can provide some added security for those with sensory or mobility impairments.

It is both fortunate from the psychological point of view and reasonable that over 60 percent of elderly and handicapped people in the United States live in cities (Golant, 1979). The stereotypical picture of older people in America assumes that they all have similar interests, health problems, financial situations, attitudes, social needs, and so on. Carp (1976) notes, however, that as people live longer, they become more diverse, not more similar, because of the different experiences of each. The urban environment usually provides a greater variety of stimulating experiences to meet their varying needs. There is also a broader range of social services available in cities, but Flemming (1972) found a poor level of awareness among elderly and handicapped citizens regarding the kinds of financial, medical, and social aid available to them. One solution to this lack of awareness would be a systematic effort by a friend or other concerned person to contact municipal agencies or an independent living center for information. Another would be to use an occupational therapist as a consultant on self-care, home management, and environmental barriers, who would set up efficient procedures and recommend changes in the daily routine and the home environment (Maguire, 1979). Possible changes could include involvement in a senior citizen activity center, home health care for specific services (see Chapter 7), or meals-on-wheels. Participation in some sort of social service provision or hobby may or may not provide extra income, but the experience will be stimulating and beneficial in any case (Flemming, 1972). Such activities have been found to significantly delay the mental decline associated with aging and to foster the sense of dignity and independence needed for continued living in a noninstitutional setting (Carp, 1976; Maguire, 1979).

GENERAL MODIFICATIONS

Because of the infinite variety of possible combinations of physical impairments, even a home designed to be accessible will almost always require at least a few modifications or additions to maximize its utility for the new occupant. The vast majority of homes in the United States fall far short of having the minimum accessibility features necessary for meeting the needs of even moderately physically impaired people. In order to facilitate the planning of modification, this section will discuss particular rooms and areas in the typical home. It is most valuable to have some sketches of the house floor plan drawn by the occupant or a friend (not a professional), so that all changes under consideration can be carefully considered before the first nail is driven or the first board is cut. This will avoid the many complications that arise if construction is begun without adequate preparation. Finally, a relative or friend should be used as a volunteer observer throughout the project to check every modification for compliance with the original instructions (Cary, 1978). What may seem to be unimportant details to a nondisabled contractor or carpenter often prove to be critical when viewed from the position of someone using a wheelchair or a cane. To avoid misunderstandings and additional costs, it is imperative to have all agreements and plans in writing prior to beginning construction.

**Outdoors**   Proceeding in logical order from the time of arrival at one's home, the first concern is parking and unloading. A covered area at least 4 feet wider than a standard garage or carport is needed to provide room to maneuver a wheelchair while remaining protected from the weather. Somewhat less clearance is needed for crutches or a cane, but extra space is very convenient. There should also be an unobstructed path to a ramp leading to a door, with a 5-foot by 5-foot flat landing if any turns are required. If the local weather includes frequent rain, snow, or ice, the entire ramp should be covered with a roof to reduce the chances of slipping.

The ramp should conform to the standard rise of 1 foot for each 12 feet of length, if possible, even if doubling back or extra turns are needed to gain the extra length (see Figure 10.1). For most purposes wooden ramps are easier to build and are preferable, unless the elevation of the house is small, which would facilitate concrete or metal construction. The ramp should be supported by 4-inch by 4-inch posts, with 2-inch by 6-inch supports underneath. It can be covered by 1-inch by 6-inch boards (placed not more than one-quarter inch apart) to allow for drainage. An alternative covering for the ramp is 1-inch thick marine plywood, which is quicker to build with, but drains less well and costs about the same. All the lumber and supports should be of pres-

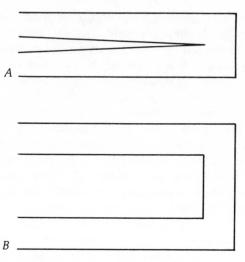

**Figure 10.1** *(A) Double-back ramp, (B) U-shaped ramp.*

sure-treated wood to inhibit rotting. The entire ramp could also be built of redwood, which lasts well but is usually more expensive. The ramp should have handrails 30 inches high made of 2-inch by 4-inch boards, with a second rail about 18 inches above the ramp surface. A strip of 1-inch by 2-inch or 2-inch by 2-inch wood should be nailed along the edges of the ramp to prevent a wheelchair's small front wheels from rolling off the surface. The top and middle rails should be at least 1½ inches from the nearest wall to allow gripping room. Wooden ramps should have some type of nonslip surface. This can be achieved by sprinkling sand on the paint while it is wet, by applying inexpensive strips of nonslip material available at most hardware stores, or by covering with a rubber surface. If a concrete ramp is built, the surface should be left rough to provide good traction.

An optional outdoor modification that this author finds very desirable is the construction of a wooden deck at the back of the house. This can be attached to the ramp near the back door or built between the door and the ramp and used as a landing area. A deck of this kind provides access to the outside when ground conditions would prohibit movement by someone who uses a wheelchair or has other mobility impairments. It can provide a useful recreation area regardless of weather conditions. The part nearest the house can have a roof over it for protection, while the rest can be uncovered for basking in the sun or viewing the stars. Attaching the deck to the rear of the house provides more privacy, and there is usually less disturbing street noise.

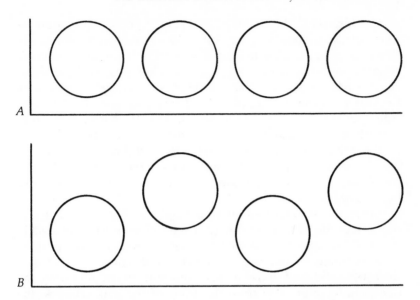

*Figure 10.2   Preferred arrangements for stovetop burners: (A) straight line, (B) staggered.*

**Kitchen**   When the arrangement of the three most used items in the kitchen—the stove, the refrigerator, and the sink—is considered, it is usually recommended that they be placed in either a U-shaped or an L-shaped pattern for maximum maneuverability ("The Accessible Home," 1981). For convenience and safety, the stove burners should be located on a countertop in either a staggered or straight line arrangement (see Figure 10.2). They should also have front controls to prevent burns (Hale, 1979). Because the standard oven door opens down, it is difficult to reach into the oven from a sitting position. A wall-mounted oven with a side-hinged door is usually recommended to avoid this problem ("The Accessible Home," 1981). Another alternative is a convection oven placed on a small table of appropriate height. These ovens are not expensive—they cost about $150—and they reduce cooking time by a third by using fan-forced heat circulation. A microwave oven is another popular choice, but even the least expensive models will cost about twice as much as a convection oven. The refrigerator should have side-by-side doors to reduce aisle blockage and make both compartments more accessible. If desired, a small portable unit can be used for frequently needed items or can be teamed with a small oven to set up a breakfast center in another room (such as the bedroom) for convenience.

Other useful appliances include a dishwasher and a trash

compactor, with the dishwasher being especially important in terms of the time and energy saved. If a garbage disposal can be fitted so as not to obstruct the sink, it, too, is useful. When considering laundry appliances, the best choice is the apartment-sized washer and dryer that are designed to stack one on top of the other. These can be placed side by side and, if they have side-opening doors, are quite easy to operate. Here again, controls should be located within easy reach, not on the back of the machine top. For those few clothes that still require ironing, a travel iron is usually best, because of its reduced weight. A small travel-size ironing board is adequate, or one can use a table with a heat-resistant surface.

Since the standard countertop height is 36 inches, 2 inches more than the 34-inch maximum height for wheelchair accessibility, it is advisable to raise the kitchen floor level. This can be done with a framework of 2-inch by 3-inch boards covered with 1-inch thick plywood and a tile or linoleum surface. By removing the doors and center strip from the front of the sink cabinets, the basins can usually be made wheelchair-accessible. In order to prevent accidental burns, the hot water pipe and the drain pipes should be wrapped with insulating material. Devices can be attached to the sink to aid the person who has full leg braces. These use straps to secure the person, and they provide balance and prevent the person from falling while using both hands in the sink. A single-lever-type water faucet should be located at one side of the sink, or, at least, not more than 21 inches from the front of the counter for use from a wheelchair. If the sink is more than 5 inches deep, racks can be placed in the bottom of each basin to raise the height to within reach. Any drain plugs should be attached to the base of the faucet with bead chains to keep them from falling out of reach and to obviate reaching into hot water to pull the plugs out.

While raising the kitchen floor will make the counter accessible, the cabinets above it are virtually useless for someone in a wheelchair. To gain maximum use of the lower cabinet space, replace the shelves with side-out drawers or revolving trays. Extra workspace can be created by installing pull-out lapboards in several places along the counter. A clearance of about 30 inches is required under these lapboards for wheelchair arms. Pans and utensils can be hung on the end of the counter and on the backs of the cabinet doors, with additional pegboard placed in a convenient location on the wall. If a utility room is connected to the kitchen, narrow shelves can be placed on the walls to provide extra storage for canned goods and other items. Pegboard can be used here for more hanging space. If any items are stored above head level, they should be lightweight enough so that one will not be injured if they fall. Any use of the higher cabinets should be aided by a reaching device, even if the person is not in a wheelchair. This will eliminate the use of footstools, which are a major source of accidents among elderly people.

**Bathroom**   Providing access to the bathroom for disabled people is a problem in most American homes because many bathrooms have doors that are narrower than standard room doorways. This problem is compounded by the fact that a straight entry into the bathroom, which is the method requiring the least clearance, is usually impossible because hallways are less than the ideal width of 48 inches (Cary, 1978). The simplest modification is using step-back hinges, which allow the door to fold back completely out of the opening, thus giving an extra inch or two of clearance (Laurie, 1977). If this is not sufficient, the doorway can be widened and extra space gained inside the bathroom by hinging the door to swing outward when opened. Once inside the bathroom, a person in a wheelchair should have an unobstructed space at least five feet in diameter for easy maneuvering. A person with good upper body strength could reduce the space needed by transferring to a smaller chair made for use in bathrooms. This would reduce or eliminate major costs associated with moving some of the fixtures, a modification that is often required in homes not constructed to be accessible. Otherwise, if the sink and toilet are on the same wall, four feet of space are needed between them for transfer to the toilet. There should be firmly anchored grab bars at the toilet, with the top of the bars being 33 inches high. A removable toilet seat extender can be added to raise the height of the seat to the recommended 19 inches (Cary, 1978). If a new toilet is purchased, one might consider a model with warm water rinsing and air drying capabilities for convenience and sanitation (Laurie, 1977).

The sink should have a height of no more than 34 inches, a single lever for controlling water flow and. temperature, and a chain attached to the drain plug, if one is used. Newer model sinks with a shallower contour, designed for use specifically by people in wheelchairs, are available ("The Accessible Home," 1981). If the bathroom has a built-in vanity, it possibily can be made accessible by removing the center doors and partition, as with the kitchen sink. The same height and clearance measurements should be used. The hot water and drain pipes should either be relocated to one side to provide knee clearance or else well insulated to prevent leg burns from accidental contact. A towel bar should be located within reach of the sink. Above the typical sink is a medicine cabinet, which is useless to a person in a wheelchair because it is out of reach. It is also too high for the mirror on its front to be useful. The best alternative is to place a long, narrow cabinet below it with sliding mirrors for doors, so that a separate cabinet is available to the disabled person. If there is a vanity in the bathroom, the side drawers that were not removed can be used for storage, and a mirror can be attached to the wall at the correct level or else mounted to triangular shims to tilt it downward for use by the person in the wheelchair.

There are a number of alternatives for bathing arrangements, depending on whether the house has a tub or a shower. For elderly people and others who are unsteady on their feet, an inexpensive nonslip surface should be applied to the tub or shower floor to prevent slips and falls. Grab bars, installed at 33 inches off the floor, may be used by disabled or elderly people for support. Both wall-mounted and tub-mounted rails are available, starting at about $20.00; price depends on the size and shape of the device (*Sears Roebuck Home Health Care Catalog*, 1981). Tub use is facilitated for disabled people by a bench that attaches across the tub and can be transferred onto easily. This type of bench can be used in conjunction with a hand-held shower unit for greater flexibility in bathing. For those who need more help, medical supply houses or department stores such as Sears can provide information on hydraulic lifts for moving from a wheelchair to the tub (Laurie, 1977).

Many advances have been made in recent years for those disabled people who prefer to bathe in the shower. It is now possible to obtain a shower that has either a small ramp on the outside and inside or a gentle slope from the floor level down into the shower unit. Both designs prevent the spillage of water onto the bathroom floor, which was a common problem with older models built level with the floor for accessibility ("The Accessible Home," 1981). One can either use a portable seat in the shower or get a shower model with a foldout seat, which can be raised out of the way when nondisabled people are bathing. The same single-lever water control is recommended here as on the sinks. To control water temperature precisely and prevent possible burns, a thermostat should be installed on the shower or tub (Hale, 1979; "The Accessible Home," 1981).

**Bedroom** Since the standard modern bed is not the correct height for transfer from a wheelchair, a platform bed is usually recommended because it can be built up to the most convenient height. One must be sure that the toeboard is recessed adequately if this option is chosen ("The Accessible Home," 1981). A cheaper alternative is to raise a standard bed to the correct height using large wooden blocks with holes for the bed legs in the tops that prevent the bed from slipping off. The same type of blocks are often used for desks and other furniture that must be raised a few inches. The headboard height should be checked, since it must be high enough to give back support when one is sitting up in bed and yet low enough to be used as a grab bar when one is transferring into bed or moving around in bed. To keep the weight of the covers off the feet so that one can turn over more easily, a U-shaped wooden piece the width of the bed is often placed at the foot of the bed, with one side of the piece slid under the mattress. The other side sticks up a few inches in the air, and the bed covers are draped over it before being tucked under.

Many of the other modifications for the bedroom are applicable to the rest of the house also. Outlets should be placed at least 18 inches from the floor to facilitate use from a wheelchair. Ideally, light switches should be 42 inches from the floor, but a flat strip of wood or plastic with a slot cut out near one end can be used to operate light switches that are too high, thus saving the expense of lowering them (Hale, 1979). Table lamps beside the bed should have either a line cord switch or a switch at the headboard. The other room lights should also have switches that can be operated from the bed. A strip with several outlets, which can be obtained at most hardware stores, is useful at the headboard, enabling one to operate extra lights or small electric appliances without having to get up to plug each one into a wall outlet.

In no other room except the kitchen is storage space as important as in the bedroom. Since most closets are considerably wider than their door openings, much of their space is unreachable from a wheelchair. The best solution is to widen the doorway and use either louvered folding doors or drawback draperies to provide easy access and yet maintain privacy. Closet rods should be placed no more than 48 inches high to be reachable. The only shelf that will probably be useful from a wheelchair is the one just above the clothes rod, and there will be little useful space below the clothes, since items on the floor cannot easily be reached. For a few dollars, shoes can be stored in a wall-hung rack on one end of a closet or on the back of a door (Hale, 1979). Purses, hats, and so on, can be placed on a shelf (at least 16 inches high) under one end of the clothes rod, with ties and belts hanging on the wall beside the rod. Extra storage space is usually desirable to replace that lost on the top closet shelves, and this can be achieved without great expense. A unit that can be moved or rearranged easily can be built by stacking various storage cubes to form the desired shape. Another alternative is a built-in bookcase or a wall unit of similar design, which can be fitted with sliding panels or drawstring draperies for privacy ("The Accessible Home," 1981).

**Miscellaneous** In addition to the individual room modifications, a number of more general features should be considered before buying or remodeling a home. Many of the more minor but still useful changes, such as the best shape of doorknobs (lever type) or the various styles and uses of reaching devices, will not be discussed, since they are thoroughly covered in most of the books referred to in this chapter. This section will focus on the more extensive and costly modifications that have general applicability to disabled or elderly people.

Concerning structural alterations of the house, there are usually several choices available in each situation. For example, if the hallways are 36 inches wide instead of the recommended 48 inches, adequate entry room can be gained by widening doorways to 36 inches. If anyone in the home uses a wheelchair, all doors should be fitted with kickplates on both sides to protect the finish from scarring by the footrests. With regard to floor surfaces, most experts recommend either hard-surface flooring or commercial-type carpeting, not the deep-pile or shag type, which are harder to roll on and may trip people who walk with difficulty. While not as easily cleaned, carpet is warmer and not as slippery as hard-surface flooring when liquids are spilled on it. A final modification concerns windows, which are a major source of problems in many homes. The most common style, double-hung, are the worst, because they are hard to operate under the best of conditions and tend to stick ("The Accessible Home," 1981). The best choice is aluminum sliding windows because they are lightweight and easy to open. All windows should start at less than 36 inches from the floor so that one can conveniently look out of them from a wheelchair (Cary, 1978).

Furniture for the home of a disabled person must be carefully chosen to fit the needs of that person. As an illustration, a disabled person would find a pedestal table with a height of at least 28 inches and a width of 42 inches or less more useful than a traditional four-legged model or a pedestal table with a smaller diameter, because it gives more footroom for the wheelchair. However, a person who might use a table for support when rising from a chair would find a pedestal table less stable than a traditional four-legged model ("The Accessible Home," 1981). Disabled people find that having smooth-rolling casters on the legs of furniture makes it easier for them to move the furniture out of the way when they want to clean the floor or retrieve dropped items. Lighter weight furniture is preferred for the same reasons. Elderly people and those with less severe mobility impairments should avoid swivel rockers and other unstable furniture (such as that on casters), using instead chairs with firm arms for support when they sit down or get up (Cary, 1978). If furniture is too low for comfortable sitting, or for transferring into, the legs can be raised using blocks with holes in the top, as described in the section on the bedroom. With regard to decoration, all mirrors and pictures should be placed at the eye level of the homeowner. If turning the standard lamp switches is difficult for someone with weak or uncoordinated fingers, the switches should be replaced with line cord switches or push-pin types.

## HEALTH AND SAFETY

Health and safety in the home take on even greater importance when the homeowner is disabled or elderly. Members of either group are likely to be more sensitive to extremes of temperature. This is especially true of elderly people because of the diminished functioning of their body temperature control mechanisms (Carp, 1976). For those who are subject to hypothermia, the preferred system of heating is one with automatic temperature control and floor or lower-wall air flow. Heat generated from the ceiling has been found to be much less satisfactory because it leaves floors and lower portions of a room too cold for people who are inactive and spend much of their time sitting (Rose, 1978). Prior to the first winter in a new location, someone should inspect the insulation level and check for air leakage around windows and doors, since many elderly and disabled people cannot do this for themselves and yet cannot afford excessive heating bills. This service can often be obtained free of charge from the local utility company by submitting a request over the phone.

Because of the reduced sensitivity of some disabled people to environmental stimuli and their impaired ability to react quickly in an emergency, safety is a critical consideration (Carp, 1976). Beginning at the outside of the home, as was done in considering structural modifications, one should make certain there is more than one accessible entrance and exit if at all possible. The area outside the home should be well-lighted, with inside and outside switches, to prevent accidents and to discourage intruders. There should also be a speaker and call button connected to an intercom system in the home so that two-way communication is possible even if one cannot get to the door. Systems that include several room speakers and a speaker for outdoors are available for about $250 or less (*J. C. Penney Catalog*, 1981). For the peace of mind of people who live in high-crime areas, burglar alarms are available from most hardware and department stores as well as from security system companies.

Since fire in the kitchen is one of the most common types of home accident, most safety experts recommend that both fire and smoke alarms be placed in the home ("The Accessible Home," 1981). The sensitivity settings on these alarms can be adjusted so that a little cooking smoke (doesn't everyone burn something occasionally?) does not trigger the mechanism. Having a small fire extinguisher is an excellent idea if one can operate it efficiently, but otherwise it may be merely a temptation to delay one's exit and thus can lead to the risk of serious injury. To help prevent cooking burns, the General Electric Company will provide knobs with braille markings for their kitchen stoves free of charge for people with visual impairments. This company will also supply cassette tapes on appliance use and care in lieu of its printed owner's manuals (Cary, 1978).

Another common type of kitchen accident among elderly people, falling off stools, can be avoided by not using the top shelves of the cabinets for anything heavy. For a few dollars, the elderly or disabled person can purchase a reacher and can then safely remove and replace lightweight items on the upper shelves (Hale, 1979).

Although the remainder of the house presents fewer safety hazards than the kitchen, with all of its appliances and activities, there are several remaining important safety checks. In the bathroom all grab bars, tub seats, seat extenders, and so on, must be firmly anchored to support repeated stress from weight bearing ("The Accessible Home," 1981). This advice includes the sink if it is ever leaned on as a person changes positions or transfers. There should be an intercom in the bathroom, so that help can be summoned quickly in case of a fall or other accident. There should also be an intercom in the bedroom, as well as a smoke alarm, especially if the battery charger for a power wheelchair is operated there or if several electrical appliances are used.

As for general safety features for the entire house, in addition to the intercom, there are several significant items. There should be no steps in the house, if possible, and if there is a single step anywhere it should be replaced with a gently sloping ramp to prevent falls. One of the most important safety devices in any emergency can be a telephone equipped with single push-button dialing. With this feature, a single preset button can be pressed and the doctor, police, fire department, or a neighbor will be called. Other special telephone adaptations for disabled people are available. The local telephone company should be contacted for details concerning services available in your area. Another possibility is a system that is connected to a hospital or medical center. In this system, which is primarily for people in poor health who live alone, a device is set to activate at two predetermined times each 24 hours. If the person does not reset the device at the prearranged times, it will automatically alert the medical facility with which it is connected. The facility then notifies a friend or neighbor who can arrive at the house in less than ten minutes and investigate the problem. Information on one such system is available from Lifeline Systems, Inc., 51 Spring Street, Watertown, Mass. 02172.

## MOBILE HOME OWNERSHIP

For those who desire the advantages of home ownership, such as income tax reductions and freedom to permanently remodel as they wish, but lack the financial resources to purchase or maintain a house, buying a mobile home is an attractive alternative. The very fact that one-half of all single-family homes purchased in the United States in 1977 were "manufactured housing" units attests to the relative attractiveness of the product (Hale, 1979). No doubt part of this sales figure reflects the growing cost of traditional housing, but the advent of larger sizes, double-wide units, and more aesthetically pleasing designs has improved both the image and the function of manufactured housing units. At this point an evaluation of the advantages, disadvantages, and location alternatives for mobile homes is in order.

### ADVANTAGES

One of the chief advantages of a mobile home for a disabled person is the ease with which it can be modified to meet accessibility standards. Many manufacturers offer units that are designed to be accessible; but if one prefers, for a small charge the company will modify the floorplan of a home before its construction—somewhat like special-ordering a car, but with greater flexibility. The manufacturer will usually change the location of doors, the width of hallways, the shape or size of rooms, and sometimes even the basic length of the unit (Laurie, 1977). For a small price it will also allow alteration or substitution of furniture to meet the needs of the buyer (Hale, 1979). The manufactured home has, of course, the same possibilities for interior design modifications after purchase as the regular home, so these will not be listed again.

The foremost advantage of manufactured housing usually cited by disabled or elderly people is, naturally, the lower purchase price and maintenance costs as compared to other homes. If a person has not previously owned a home, this smaller initial cost eases the difficulty of entering the housing market. The advantage is probably even greater for the person who has a home already, but is in a financial bind. The other home can be sold and the proceeds used to buy a manufactured home, probably without a mortgage or, at least, with only a small monthly payment. If there are any profits, they can be invested or saved to provide future security as supplementary income or to pay off medical or other expenses. In some states mobile homes are also taxed as vehicles rather than as property, resulting in a substantial savings to the owner.

## DISADVANTAGES

As in many purchases with a lower initial cost, the mobile home has several "hidden" costs that may not be apparent to the first-time buyer. The most subtle of these is depreciation, which is just the opposite of the customary gradual increase in the value of the traditional home (Laurie, 1977). Just as with standard housing, this problem is worse if the unit is poorly constructed or located in a depressed area, but depreciation does affect all units to some degree. Before buying the unit, one should find out (in writing) exactly what installation services are free and what other required services would cost if performed by the dealer. Additional expenses include installation of utilities, cost of underpinning, and rental of a lot if the land is not already owned by the home buyer. One should also find out the insulation specifications of the particular unit, because some units are insulated differently, depending on the region of the United States where they will be sold. To avoid exorbitant utility bills, the maximum insulation and a concrete block underpinning are recommended in all but the warmest parts of the country.

## MANUFACTURED HOUSING LOCATION OPTIONS

As is the case with regular housing, the urban setting is usually preferable for any disabled person who may need regular medical or social services; it also provides more social stimulation, which has been found to be beneficial (Carp, 1976; Hasselkus and Kiernat, 1973). Before choosing any site for a mobile home, one should contact the mobile home (or manufactured housing) association in the state of prospective residence. This organization can usually supply a list of parks in the state and their ratings, which are important for both social and financial reasons, as discussed in the previous section. A suitable lot should be located, community services investigated, and financing considered before the home is bought. Some of the better parks for mobile homes provide garbage service, laundry facilities, and social and recreational facilities (Laurie, 1977).

All of the above discussion assumes that the new mobile home owner will have to rent a lot on which to park the home. If the person already owns some real estate that is zoned for mobile homes, there are some different factors to consider. Instead of lot rental fees, the owner will have either property taxes or vehicle taxes to pay, the latter being much less. The cost of property taxes is reduced somewhat by the fact that they are income-tax deductible. If the land one owns already has utilities, one can probably connect to the existing lines, if the local authorities approve. If some or all utilities are missing, the home's initial installation cost will be greater and there may be some delay. Before making any plans or purchases, it is wise to contact the city or county zoning commission to determine the zoning and construction restrictions of the property, including such items as type of underpinning or foundation materials required. Despite the former name "mobile homes," statistics show that only 10 percent of the manufactured housing units sold are ever moved after the initial set-up, so any location that is chosen must be considered as likely to be the permanent site. This should induce caution on the part of the disabled or elderly buyer (Laurie, 1977).

## APARTMENT RENTAL

Although renting one's own apartment does not involve the same financial commitment that buying a home or a mobile home does, it is similar in terms of the physical independence achieved and the psychological preparation and commitment required. The fact that the disabled renter is living and functioning outside an institutional environment and is responsible for all of the daily decisions of life is both comforting and anxiety-provoking. Within this context there are a number of options available, which allows the disabled person to select the living situation most compatible with his or her needs.

Because of the lower amount of cash required and the fact that the renter is not responsible for maintenance, renting an apartment is a viable alternative for disabled people seeking independence. Even up until the early 1970s, most of the accessible apartments in the United States were to be found in complexes where all of the units were specially designed for use by disabled or elderly tenants exclusively, while in some European countries, such as Sweden and Holland, housing for disabled citizens was being integrated into the general community (Greenstein, Gueli, and Leonard, 1976). The segregation of housing for the disabled and elderly in America contributed to a somewhat less than desirable image for these complexes among their targeted groups. Among people who were very conscious of independence, these complexes were sometimes accepted with the same enthusiasm as the "separate but equal" doctrine was among minorities, because the very fact of segregation inherently implied an undesirable distinction. This attitude toward accessible housing is no longer necessarily justified, because some complexes serving special populations now are fine facilities and offer attractive accommodations. The rental rates are sometimes slightly lower, too. If such apartments are available in the prospective area of residence, they should be investigated with an open mind.

Nevertheless, the desire of many disabled people to live and function in regular apartment complexes for the nondisabled is still strong. In recognition of this desire, some building contractors are now including in their apartment buildings a few units that are adapted to the needs of disabled people or elderly people with mobility impairments. These units are financially profitable because there is usually sufficient demand for such housing to ensure high occupancy rates. The remainder of this section will focus primarily on these apartments, since specialized complexes usually have staffs to provide many services to tenants that would usually be the responsibility of the individual (Laurie, 1977). The discussion will consider the advantages and disadvantages of apartment living, as well as possible modifications to the premises.

## ADVANTAGES

While the most obvious advantage of an apartment for anyone, disabled or not, is the absence of a large down payment, closing costs, and other expenses associated with buying a dwelling, apartment living also has real social advantages for disabled and elderly people. In contrast to the isolation that is common among homeowners, apartment dwellers are in a natural setting for interaction and can take advantage of the everyday contacts that occur between residents. Many complexes provide laundry facilities and recreation areas, and a few have eating facilities (May et al., 1974). Usually apartments are located near shopping centers, public transportation, and entertainment, and this creates further opportunities for pleasurable experiences and new friends (Cary, 1978). Rose (1978) found that in recognition of interpersonal needs, some apartment complexes even have multipurpose rooms that, with advance notice, are converted to guest rooms. This encourages visitors to come and spend more time with tenants than if they had to stay in a hotel some distance away. This especially helps elderly disabled tenants not yet accustomed to the new environment.

Apartment living also avoids many of the routine problems, such as repairs and maintenance of the property, that disabled people associate with home ownership. The tenant does not have to worry about cutting the grass, painting the walls, or fixing leaky faucets, because these and similar jobs are handled by the management. Most modern apartments also have central heating and air conditioning with individual controls for each apartment. In some private apartments arrangements can even be made for services that tenants need, such as health care, social services, homemaker aides, or other special assistance, but this is usually true only in complexes restricted to elderly or disabled people (Laurie, 1977). Newcomer (1976) notes that 12 percent of elderly people need some kind of support service to live independently, and he estimates that the percentage is as high as 20 percent among elderly poor people. In apartment buildings occupied primarily by nondisabled, younger people, there are usually enough disabled or elderly tenants needing particular services, such as cleaning, transportation, or attendant care, to enable them to combine their needs and construct a schedule. Then they can retain one or more people on a fulltime basis without paying exorbitant prices. The employed people are happier also because they can work full time in one location, rather than traveling to several sites, as they would have to do with individual home-owners. Laurie (1977) notes that some nursing homes now provide a similar service by locating mobile home communities next to the nursing home buildings. These units are rented under a plan similar to independent apartments, but with extra services. The nursing home switchboard is connected to each mobile home, providing 24-hour-a-day access to nursing and medical help. This arrangement provides an alternative for people who wish to live independently but who may have difficulties that need medical supervision. These homes also frequently have a meal plan, so that those who live in the mobile homes can eat in the dining facility on the nursing home grounds if they wish.

## DISADVANTAGES

For a disabled person there are two major drawbacks to renting an apartment. First, there is the standard lease, which may be for six months, but is usually for a one-year minimum, and which is expensive to break if the person rents an inappropriate unit and must move early. Second, there is the fact that if the unit is not exactly suited to the person's needs, it cannot be permanently modified, except possibly in minor ways approved by the management. In many apartment buildings, disabled residents find problems with the windows, cupboards, bathrooms, hall lighting, and ventilation, so these areas in particular should be investigated for suitability or ease of use before a rental contract is signed (Rose, 1978). Another problem, which most affects elderly disabled people, is inadequate sound insulation (Carp, 1976). Research has shown that background noise is not as easily screened out by the auditory system of older people and can cause confusion and irritability, which is certainly undesirable in a place of long-term residence. A final consideration is that if one rents an unsuitable apartment and complains too frequently, he or she may face eviction and suddenly be homeless.

## APARTMENT MODIFICATIONS

The most obvious characteristics required of alterations in a rented apartment are that they must be temporary and nondamaging to the unit. Some of the adaptations suggested for the home can be used in apartments, such as removable toilet seat extenders, tub benches, and a hand-held shower attachment. In the kitchen one can add a tier of hanging vegetable baskets to the end of the cabinets to raise vegetables to a reachable height and save floor space. Reachers, blocks under the legs of too-short furniture, and devices for reaching wall switches can all still be used. If an electrically operated hospital-type bed is needed, some units available from department stores can be placed onto regular bed frames, and their cost is well below that of a full hospital bed unit (*Sears Roebuck Home Health Care Catalog*, 1981). Most of the other interior modifications listed earlier that do not involve cutting or moving structural materials can be incorporated, but one should consult the building manager before proceeding to make changes.

There are a few changes suited to apartments that have not been listed earlier. If the apartment floor plan includes a small difference in floor levels (one step or less), a portable or temporary ramp can be used as a solution. To compensate for unusable closet space, a wardrobe unit with either sliding or regular hinged doors can be purchased from major department stores for about $100–150. The clothes rod in these units is usually already at an accessible height. Other changes, such as removing closet or bathroom doors and installing fold-back hinges, may be permissible, but should be approved by management.

## SUMMARY

Choosing a place of residence is one of the most serious decisions anyone can undertake, because of its influence on so much of one's life. The importance of a choice of residence is multiplied for the disabled person who has limited physical, financial, or social resources and who thus may be even more affected by the place of residence. As noted by Lifchez and Winslow (1979), independence is a state of mind. It is a determination to accomplish those things that the individual considers important, making whatever adjustments are necessary in life or lifestyle to reach those goals. This kind of attitude is not dependent on dusting one's own furniture or owning a home, but on the selection of, and dedication to, one's own priorities. An ill-conceived attempt to live alone in one's own house without needed medical or home care services may impair one's health (and ultimate independence) as much as being unnecessarily confined in a restrictive institutional setting.

Before any decision is made about moving into a house, mobile home, or apartment, the disabled person must take an honest inventory of how his or her abilities and handicaps relate to various living situations. This cannot usually be done alone with completely realistic results, so advice should be sought from people with experience in the area and no vested interest in one's choice. The effects of any particular mobility impairment can be evaluated at a local independent living center, if one is available. Other professional advice could be obtained from an occupational or physical therapist, or a vocational evaluation specialist in a rehabilitation center.

Two final factors that must be taken into account before any decision on living arrangements is made are money and location. In addition to down payment or deposit, monthly payment or rent, and utilities, most disabled people will face some extra expenses related to modifications. In order to gain some accurate idea of the probable costs of changes, one should visit several prospective locations, preferably accompanied by a carpenter or someone with a knowledge of material and construction costs. A low purchase price or rent is worthless if one cannot afford the accessibility modifications that are required. Even if no important changes are needed, one must also investigate the neighborhood for safety, convenience to shopping and other services, and general desirability. In short, the disabled person must take all the normal precautions of a wise resident, but with extra attention to the alterations necessitated by his or her particular requirements. Realism is the central point in all of these considerations, so that one does not become committed to an undesirable or unhealthy situation without being able to move or correct the problems.

# 11

## Nonresidential Independent Living Centers

This chapter will present descriptive information regarding the services available through nonresidential IL centers—that is, those facilities that provide or arrange services related to daily living for disabled people but do not offer residential accommodations. IL centers, both residential and nonresidential, were established to go beyond the employment-centered concept of vocational rehabilitation and assist disabled people to develop their social skills, make better use of their leisure time, and acquire personal skills that would help them achieve greater independence (Baum, 1980). After a discussion of the kinds of services usually found in typical nonresidential IL centers, a separate section of this chapter will be devoted to those nonresidential programs with a special emphasis on disabled geriatric people and their needs. Both the day hospital and the community-based geriatric treatment approaches described in that section are viable lower-cost alternatives to institutional or home-bound care for a significant number of elderly people.

## TRADITIONAL INDEPENDENT LIVING PROGRAMS

As noted in previous chapters, the definition of independent living is not the same for every disabled person, but varies with the individual's needs, goals, and personal priorities. How one lives will have an influence on how one carries out the activities of daily living and on what services one needs from an IL center. In spite of the wide range of services required by different disabled people, Stoddard and Brown (1980) found that California's 11 IL centers were meeting over 75 percent of all client needs. It appears from their survey results, and an extensive review of other centers by this author, that there is a great similarity in the services offered at most centers. Services in the following categories have been found to be widely available and will be discussed in some detail: housing; independent living skills training; attendants; mobility; peer counseling; professional counseling; communications; social and recreational, vocational, and consumer-oriented services (ILRUP, 1979). These services are all either mandated by the 1978 Amendments to the Rehabilitation Act of 1973 or else are supplementary to those mandated services. The number and variety of services provided within each category will vary from center to center. Whether a particular service is provided directly or through referral to other sources depends on the center's philosophy, size, and financial condition. The information given here is intended as a comprehensive general guide. Information as to exactly what services a particular center offers should be obtained through local agencies.

### HOUSING SERVICES

Because of the financial costs and the multitude of complicated regulations involved in establishing and operating a residential facility, most IL centers are nonresidential in nature (ILRUP, 1979). They assist disabled people to achieve or maintain the ability to live and function independently in the community. Their primary involvement in housing is in providing a register of accessible accommodations. This register should include both apartments and private homes. A register of private homes, however, is often difficult to establish without a community-wide survey such as the "Access 80s" program being conducted in Memphis by the Easter Seal Center for Independent Living. Centers can also involve themselves with housing by sponsoring shared-housing programs in which two or more interested people are brought together and helped to locate and rent or purchase a suitable house or apartment. Sometimes in these programs one or more of the residents is not disabled and will perform some attendant duties as part of his or her occupancy agreement, thus reducing the disabled person's need for outside attendants.

Housing opportunities for physically handicapped people began increasing in 1965, when they were included with the elderly under the Section 202 regulations (Ross, 1980). This legislation provided for assistance with housing construction and with substantial rehabilitations of existing housing. Major improvements in housing access came as a result of the passage of Public Law 93-383, the Housing and Community Development Act of 1974. Section 235 of this law provides home ownership assistance, while Section 8 deals with rental subsidies, moderate or substantial home rehabilitation, new construction, and mortgage insurance protection. The rent subsidies can be used not only in public housing but even for a unit one already occupies, upon proper application to HUD (Harwell, 1980). Under both Sections 8 and 235, a disabled person is considered a "family" for purposes of eligibility. Most IL centers should have, or be able to obtain, a list of local housing units that qualify for these programs, as well as the guidelines for individual eligibility. These centers are often a good source of information on housing modifications, and may sponsor housing workshops utilizing community professionals such as building contractors, architects, and so on. Many centers will even arrange for an occupational therapist or other qualified rehabilitation specialist to make a home visit and suggest alterations that will make the unit more functional for the disabled person (Maguire, 1979).

## INDEPENDENT LIVING SKILL TRAINING

Almost all IL centers provide some level of IL skill training within their program, although some either provide referral to another agency or arrange for the client to contact a therapist. Physical or occupational therapists are especially useful to the disabled person who has limited transportation or who needs some specific suggestions regarding adaptive equipment or how to modify an unsatisfactory dwelling. Home visits by either a staff member or a therapist are usually arranged only when the center receives a direct request from a client or a referring agency. Consultation with a therapist is also useful when a client needs someone to recommend alternative ways of performing particular activities, such as transferring or dressing, when the standard methods are not possible because of a loss of muscle strength or other physical problem. Sometimes a center will be able to refer the disabled person to a community volunteer program that has a list of helpers who are available at various times to provide help with household or personal tasks.

Nonresidential centers that do provide in-house IL skill training will have at least one full-time counselor on the staff who can give professional advice and personal assistance on client problems. In addition to part-time assistance from other staff members, the center will have a large complement of peer tutors who perform much of the day-to-day instruction in specific skills. The involvement of these peer tutors is very valuable because of the large amount of time that a disabled person often requires to master some IL skills. The personal experiences of these tutors with disability, and their success in overcoming its effects, not only give authenticity to their teaching, but are motivating factors as well. Well-established centers sponsor periodic workshops with community resource people, such as doctors, public health nurses, therapists, or prominent disabled business people. The emphasis in these workshops may range from introducing clients to new equipment or exercises to motivational themes or time-management practices. When they are open to the entire disabled community, such meetings provide both information to disabled people and public exposure for the center.

## ATTENDANT SERVICES

The ability of an IL center to provide the disabled person with a source of dependable, qualified attendant care is often of critical importance and is recognized as such in the 1978 Amendments to the Rehabilitation Act of 1973 (ILRUP, 1979). Without such assistance the disabled person's health will suffer and the result may be institutionalization. Smith and Meyer (1981) have documented the need for reliable personal care and the most frequent sources of problems related to attendants. Citing an average length of employment for attendants of only six months per job, they list low pay, low job status, and lack of interest in the job as the major factors producing disenchantment and turnover. These factors also contribute to the difficulty of attracting applicants of better quality, which is the root of the entire problem.

Considering the necessity of good attendant care in helping disabled people maintain their independence, morale, and physical condition, not to mention reducing their families' burdens, the role of the nonresidential IL center is very important. An active center can be a focal point for drawing community attention to the needs, and the abilities, of disabled people. The center is a natural place for the recruitment and training of good personal care attendants because of its experienced staff, especially the peer tutors, who can provide detailed information and instruction regarding the needs of its disabled clients. The IL center that provides on-site attendant training can better utilize its attendant register because the staff will be well acquainted with both the attendant and the disabled person and can better match their personalities, needs, and abilities. The center staff is also sometimes able to find another disabled person with complementary needs who can share an attendant, thus reducing each client's expense and producing more work and income for the attendant.

Many IL centers are also involved in the other side of attendant services—teaching disabled people how to manage an attendant. As pointed out by Smith and Meyer (1981), the disabled person who has an attendant is actually an employer and needs certain business knowledge. Training for attendant management includes such skills as hiring and firing, determining pay and job description, and establishing a proper working relationship. The disabled employer is taught, for example, that if his or her finances are limited, then he or she must be more selective in deciding the number of duties an attendant is to perform and the number of hours an attendant is to work. The disabled person is also cautioned against developing too close a relationship with the attendant, as this can lead to emotional conflict or dependence. To avoid the problem of rapid turnover, the IL center carefully screens the attendant applicants before and during their training. In addition to the typical use of middle-aged people seeking part-time work, some centers have had success with college students who were emotionally mature and in need of money to continue their education. Especially in hard economic times, a steady part-time job for the duration of their school years appeals to some students, while providing active, reliable care for the disabled person.

## MOBILITY SERVICES

In discussing the mobility of disabled people, a distinction emerges between personal movement and movement throughout the community. In the first type, which involves primarily the home and immediate vicinity, a wheelchair, walker, or white cane (if visually impaired) might be required. Many centers provide these kinds of items on loan for a few months without cost, until the person can choose and acquire the equipment suited to his or her particular needs. The client also can call on advice from the center staff, and other professionals if necessary, before buying such adaptive equipment. The center will provide training in the use of the new equipment or will refer the person to a community program. The Goodwill program in Memphis, which teaches visually impaired people to navigate in the city, is a good example of this kind of service.

While some large centers, such as the Center for Independent Living in Berkeley, still are able to provide transportation for their clients, many centers, for financial reasons, now restrict their direct transportation services to meeting a client's medical, therapy, or similar appointments (ILRUP, 1979). Since public transportation services in many cities now provide special vehicles or reduced fares for disabled people, IL centers primarily act as certifying agents to entitle their clients to the special benefits. Disabled people wishing to purchase a modified vehicle or install special equipment in a standard automobile can get information and counseling on such devices, including dealers' names, costs, and so on, from the center staff. Training in the use of this equipment is available from both the dealer and the center. With the cooperation of local businesses and volunteers, centers usually hold an annual repair day for wheelchairs and other mobility devices. On such occasions, labor is free and parts are provided either free or at greatly reduced cost.

PEER COUNSELING

In addition to providing information and advice regarding the selection of adaptive equipment, peer counselors offer important personal counseling services to the center's clients. Having had their own experiences with overcoming disabilities, the peer counselors frequently are instrumental in facilitating the emotional adjustment of others in similar circumstances. They are able to reassure clients that certain reactions to disability, such as depression, hostility, and guilt, are not unique to them. As the emotional aspects of the person's problems are worked out, the peer counselor is able to suggest alternative methods of coping that he or she has personally found helpful. In addition to personal counseling, peer counselors may provide clients with financial counseling and advice regarding the availability and use of community service programs (Cole, 1979). The inclusion of peer assistance in the services to be provided by approved IL centers under the 1978 Rehabilitation Amendments has ensured the connued presence of these valuable resource personnel (ILRUP, '79).

## PROFESSIONAL COUNSELING

Although professional counselors are involved in some of the same areas as peer counselors, such as facilitating emotional and sexual adjustment, they usually deal only with the more severe cases. In most centers, such as the Memphis Center for Independent Living, this is due to the limited number of professional counselors available, as compared to the number of peer counselors. In the nonresidential center, professional counselors will conduct group counseling and assertiveness training sessions, as well as handling family crisis situations. Through these services and other group projects and activities, the center attempts to provide a supportive environment for its clients.

For technical or legal matters, the client will be referred to outside professional help, such as a doctor, public health nurse, accountant, or lawyer. If the disabled person is a veteran of the armed services, excellent family counseling, health or educational benefits, or other services are available from the Veterans Administration. Similar services are also available through state vocational rehabilitation programs. When the center refers a client to any outside agency, the client should be given the name of a contact person, a list of the requirements for eligibility, and a description of the program and its purposes. This is helpful to both the client and the receiving agency. It saves time and alleviates fears and misunderstanding, as well as reducing the number of inappropriate referrals.

## COMMUNICATIONS

The fundamental worth of any IL center depends on the quantity and quality of its two-way communication with its clients. Unless both staff and clients feel free to give positive and negative feedback, as well as suggestions for change, the center will become inflexible and stagnant. For example, the presence of a telecommunications unit for use by hearing-impaired people, whether they are clients of the center or not, has both practical and psychological benefits because it reduces their feelings of being excluded. At a less personal level of communication, a newsletter has been found to be an efficient method of information exchange when it is open to contributions from both clients and people in the community, as well as from the center staff. A newsletter can function as a reference source for clients if information on upcoming legislation or civic activities is included.

Many IL centers frequently exchange information with other centers. The Memphis Center for Independent Living uses these exchanges as a source of information on new ideas and successful new services or programs. Informal links are also maintained with local hospitals and institutions of higher education. The IL center provides in-service training for personnel from hospitals, colleges, universities, and other community agencies upon request and participates in joint research projects and surveys. The center encourages utilization of its resource library by clients and community professionals. Typical materials include 16mm films, slides and cassettes, books, brochures, and the Federal Register. Information is available on other IL programs, rehabilitation engineering, and the rehabilitation of severely disabled people, as well as training materials on activities of daily living and other subjects pertinent to the disabled person's advancement toward independence. Space is made available in the center to community groups for meetings, which increases contact with, and understanding of, the center's program and the population it serves.

## SOCIAL AND RECREATIONAL SERVICES

Another way that the center can increase public awareness and acceptance of handicapping conditions while fostering independence and activity on the part of disabled people is by sponsoring social activities for its clients in the community. Common ways of doing this include field trips to local attractions and monthly outings to restaurants. IL centers can frequently obtain discount tickets to entertainment events such as concerts, plays, ballgames, and so on. Among the sponsored activities promoting fitness as well as fellowship are bowling leagues, track and field meets, wheelchair basketball teams, and marathon races. Some of the sponsored activities are not limited to center clients, but are open to all interested disabled people in the local area. Cole (1979) found that social and recreational services were provided by almost 60 percent of the IL centers surveyed. This percentage appears to be growing as the scope of services expands beyond basic necessities to include activities aimed at promoting a well-rounded lifestyle for disabled people.

## VOCATIONAL SERVICES

Besides sponsoring the educational and vocational referral services mentioned in the section of this chapter on counseling, the

IL center is involved with client vocational needs in several other ways. To prepare the client for job-seeking, the center will video-tape simulated job interviews upon request. In addition to keeping a list of clients needing employment, the center keeps a register of known jobs and maintains two-way communication with the local vocational rehabilitation office to ensure greater utilization of this information. Neither Stoddard and Brown (1980) nor Cole (1979) listed vocational services as a primary feature of IL programs in general. The ILRUP *Sourcebook* (ILRUP, 1979) did list some nonresidential IL centers with an incidental emphasis on vocational areas, but those programs with a stronger vocational emphasis were usually found in residential rehabilitation centers such as Warm Springs in Georgia. Now, however, some nonresidential centers, such as the Center for Independent Living in Memphis, are developing cooperative plans with other facilities to obtain evaluation, training, and employment services for their clients.

CONSUMER-ORIENTED SERVICES

With the emerging emphasis on the importance of a well-rounded life for disabled people, the involvement of coordinative IL centers in consumer education has increased greatly. The center originally focused on public issues such as access to treatment information, removal of architectural barriers, and legislation affecting discrimination, education, and employment. While these concerns are necessarily still prominent, attention is now also being devoted to matters of more personal relevance. IL centers now offer information or classes on the medical aspects of disability, emergency medical procedures, comparison shopping methods, the accessibility of local (and national) tourist attractions and housing accommodations, and a wide array of other subjects. Through cooperation with other centers and library information services, the IL center can assist the disabled person with almost any request for information affecting daily life.

## NONRESIDENTIAL GERIATRIC SERVICES

Although elderly disabled people are eligible for services at the nonresidential living centers described above, and many such people are served there, there are other sources of assistance specially designed to meet the differing needs of many older people. Some of their needs, such as nutritional support and regular medical examinations, are not easily supplied by the typical non-residential IL center. We will examine two kinds of nonresidential programs for elderly people: those programs that are hospital-based and those that are community-based.

## DAY HOSPITAL GERIATRIC SERVICES

A "day hospital" is described as a hospital-based facility where patients come during the day to receive therapy, medical examinations, and social, recreational, and rehabilitation services (Aronson, 1976; Matlack, 1975). Each person is also provided with a balanced lunch and has two short breaks during the four to eight hours he or she spends at the hospital. Since, on the average, clients attend only two days per week, the day hospital can serve a larger population than might be immediately apparent. The goals of the program are to discharge inpatients earlier, to reduce the need for institutionalization among elderly disabled people, and to lower the hospital readmission rate—a rate that, measured one year after the patient's initial discharge, has reached 70 percent (Matlack, 1975).

Although the day hospital concept has been in use in Europe for about thirty years, it has only been adopted on even a small scale in the United States within the last decade. Because of the definite advantages it has over both institutionalization and the home health care method, this type of program should become increasingly widespread in the United States (Brickner et al., 1976). The time spent away from home at the day hospital provides mental stimulation and social interaction, not to mention access to many more services than could usually be supplied on home visits (Novick, 1973; Williams and Benes, 1976). Not only are the geriatric services more comprehensive at the day hospital, but they are less expensive than even home health care (40 percent of inpatient costs, as compared to 50 percent of the home visit method). This is due to the elimination of staff travel and the use of small groups rather than individuals in some activities (Brickner et al., 1976; Novick, 1973).

The major day hospitals, such as Maimonides Hospital and Home for the Aged in Montreal and the Day Hospital at Burke Rehabilitation Center in White Plains, New York, are self-supporting institutions with a full complement of professional personnel. Their staff typically includes a doctor, a psychiatrist, nurses, a physical therapist, an occupational therapist, a social worker, other therapists or assistants, and a dietician (Novick, 1973; Williams and Benes, 1976). Most day hospitals have two programs, an intensive program and an intermediate one. The short-term, intensive program consists of individual sessions focused on activities of daily living, homemaking, communication and socialization skills, and the use of specialized therapy equipment. The intermediate program is designed for those who will profit from long-term, group-oriented activities. It is aimed at maintaining residual physical function and providing mental and social stimulation. Often patients move from the regular hospital to the intensive program and then into the intermediate program, but this is not a rigid procedure. Skilled nursing, rehabilitative services, and the availability of regular medical exams and treatment are central to the care of all day hospital participants (Kiernat, 1976). Other support services offered may include arts and crafts classes, planned outings, sheltered vocational work, speech therapy, dietary counseling, home visits and evaluations, and transportation (Williams and Benes, 1976).

Although the day hospital program has some obvious similarities to the programs of senior citizen centers and other recreational groups, there are some important differences. Because of the poorer state of health of the participants in day hospital programs, there is a natural emphasis on restorative services, but the atmosphere is as congenial and relaxed as possible. Second, the activities at the day hospital, unlike those of social clubs, are not designed to be self-fulfilling, but are directed primarily toward improving the ability of the person to live a healthy, happy, independent life at home. Novick (1973) notes that in the first four years of operation at Maimonides Hospital, only 6 percent of patients were placed into institutional care, which indicates that the program does work. In fact, a later followup by Aronson (1976) shows that after 10 years of operation the Maimonides Hospital had evolved to serve a broader population and was seeing so much improvement in some patients that they could be discharged. This is a pleasant and important contrast to the frequent deterioration of institutionalized elderly people.

## COMMUNITY-BASED GERIATRIC PROGRAMS

Occupational therapists or rehabilitation professionals can be very helpful to the disabled person. They can teach self-help skills, suggest home modifications and adaptive furnishings, and advise on a number of related problems. They cannot, however, be present in the home of every client on a daily basis to assist with routine tasks. In the spirit of volunteerism and social concern, various types of projects have developed spontaneously to assist disabled people, and especially the elderly disabled, with these tasks. In many communities these programs are the only help available to indigent disabled people.

Typical of more formal programs, which concentrate on teaching skills as well as providing services, was the Independent Living Project for the Elderly in Madison, Wisconsin (Hasselkus and Kiernat, 1973). This project had an Adult Education phase that covered self-care in a wheelchair, independence for one-handed people, solutions for arthritis problems, special telephone services, consumer protection, and other subjects. In Phase Two it provided home consultations, referral to a mobile meal program, home safety tips, and so on. In Phase Three regularly scheduled transportation was provided for shopping and personal business, medical appointments, and other meetings. Although it was not really comprehensive, this program contributed substantially to the ability of its participants to remain independent in their homes.

A more informal type of program is found in many communities. These programs are often sponsored by churches or neighborhood civic groups motivated by a personal knowledge of the human needs in their immediate area. They usually establish a pool of volunteers who list the hours and days they are available to provide assistance. Another register will contain the names of people who desire specific services, and, through individual contacts, a schedule of services is arranged for each disabled person. Typical volunteer services include housecleaning, cooking, personal care, and transportation. The kinds of IL skills taught depends upon the knowledge and attitude of the volunteer and the recipient. These simple programs can provide the social contact that is often missing and at the same time help the elderly disabled person retain the sense of dignity and independence that is important in forestalling institutionalization (Maguire, 1979).

# 12

## Residential Independent Living Programs

At the opposite end of the continuum from private homes and apartments are facilities known as IL residential centers and group homes. Both of these types of facilities provide a number of rehabilitation services and options to disabled people in a residential setting while still allowing a relatively autonomous lifestyle. These facilities, with their encouragement of client independence and personal growth, are a radical departure from the historical practices of warehousing and custodial supervision of disabled people. The variety of living arrangements and available services provided by modern IL centers and group homes gives the disabled person a great deal of flexibility in choosing a personally satisfying lifestyle. IL programs must continue to expand and innovate if the trend toward increased institutionalization of disabled and elderly people is to be reversed (Rabin, 1981). The resulting reduction in the number of institutionalized people will be financially and psychologically beneficial both to society and to the individuals who achieve independence.

This chapter will be divided into three sections, with the first section providing information on transitional or short-term IL

223

centers, while the second section deals with long-term residential centers. The two predominant types of group homes, single units and cluster arrangements, will be analyzed in the third section. Each type of facility will be discussed with regard to its operational philosophy and the services provided. The advantages and disadvantages of each residential model for the individual disabled resident will be considered at the end of the chapter. Direct comparisons of the various programs will be included where these are feasible and informative.

## TRANSITIONAL INDEPENDENT LIVING CENTERS

Transitional IL residential programs are described by Frieden (1980) as facilitating the progression of disabled individuals from a state of relative dependence to a state of relative independence with regard to their living situations. The transitional facility's primary goal is to enable the disabled person to reach new levels of proficiency in self-care. Thus, the primary services provided are in the form of IL skill training. The transitional IL center is usually goal- or time-oriented, having predetermined criteria regarding the desirable level of proficiency or length of residence expected of the client. By the time of the expiration of this training program, the client is prepared for graduation from the transitional center into an appropriate living situation in the community (ILRUP, 1979). The philosophy of the transitional IL centers is indicated by their concern with skill acquisition and time, which leads them to accept as clients those who are expected to progress fairly rapidly, such as recently disabled people still experiencing some medical recovery or people who need specific self-care skills. In fact, a growing number of hospitals are adding special care or extended care units to their facilities to provide the patient with some transitional rehabilitation services before discharge. Many of these units have been developed especially to serve elderly disabled people who need closer medical attention during their initial recovery from the disabling incident. Upon leaving the extended care unit, the disabled person is often referred to a transitional IL center for more comprehensive services prior to returning to the community.

### SERVICES PROVIDED

To simplify the discussion, the services usually available at transitional IL living centers will be divided into three categories: personal, social, and business-related. The method of teaching these skills varies, but most centers use either a module format or an individual evaluation procedure. Centers such as the Roosevelt Warm Springs Institute for Rehabilitation in Georgia or New Options in Houston have found it preferable to develop a somewhat standardized program of modules covering anticipated areas of client need (Cole, 1979; Roosevelt Warm Springs, 1981). These modules are all completed by each client during the six-week program and their comprehensive content minimizes the possibility—always a danger with individual evaluations—that an area of need might be overlooked. The topics presented in the modules at Roosevelt Warm Springs, New Options, and similar centers form the basis of the following discussion of IL services in a transitional residential setting. It should be noted that other transitional IL centers that have longer programs, such as the Boston Center for Independent Living, provide essentially the same services, but they do so through individualized programs (BCIL, undated).

**Personal Skills**  These are probably the most basic, and the most obvious, skills a disabled person must master to become independent. Usually functional skills and medical needs receive attention first. Functional skills include the activities of daily living, such as bathing, dressing, grooming, eating, and elimination. The client is shown alternative methods of performing each task and learns to accomplish each as independently as possible. Emphasis is placed on the kinds of medical care and their importance to health, and the proper frequency of examinations. Instruction is given in preventive self-care measures, such as checking for any redness, swelling, or bodily changes when one is bathing. Another important service is psychological counseling regarding personal adjustment, family problems, or related matters. Finally, there is now a recognition of the sexual and affection needs of disabled people, so that many centers offer both counseling and instruction on sexual matters and practices.

**Social Skills**  Classes on social skills at transitional IL centers cover a variety of subjects, including transportation, mobility, and community participation. While centers do provide some basic transportation, their primary role is to prepare the client for independent travel. Clients who have a personal vehicle are advised about the modifications or devices needed to allow its continued use, or about the purchase of an accessible vehicle. Other clients are taught to use whatever public transportation is available and to arrange for private transportation when necessary. Emphasis is also placed on the acquisition of personal mobility skills using a wheelchair, crutches, prosthesis, or other device. Mobility in the community is not the end goal, but is a means of growth in that it allows broadened experiences and interactions. Transitional residential centers arrange a variety of community experiences for clients, including social outings and recreational activities. Examples include shopping trips, dining out, nature outings, observing or participating in sports events, and learning various arts and crafts (Roosevelt Warm Springs, 1981). These experiences not only produce more well-rounded people but reduce the initial fears that often hinder disabled people from being active in the community when they leave the center. When the disabled person is ready to move out, the center provides counseling concerning what living situations would be most appropriate, and a register of apartments and homes is available to provide a starting point for the selection process.

**Business-Related Skills**   A number of business-related skills are important to the disabled person's independence. On a personal level, the typical transitional center provides counseling related to the educational and vocational opportunities open to each client. Often this includes vocational evaluation and occupational exploration under the guidance of a professional evaluator or vocational rehabilitation counselor. Examples of centers with such vocational services include The Independent Living Center (Bangor, Maine), Worcester Area Transitional Housing (Worcester, Massachusetts), and the Rehabilitation Institute–Center for Independent Living (Detroit, Michigan). The prerequisites for hiring, managing, and firing a personal care attendant are also the subject of careful instruction by the center, because of the importance of an attendant to the client's health and wellbeing. Such ordinarily routine matters as the management of one's time and money become crucial to the disabled person. With the increased time required for many routine activities and the cost of having a person employed to assist with each one, the budgeting of the disabled person's limited time and finances is a key subject for special instruction and counseling. In addition, the transitional center must promote client awareness of consumer affairs. This area includes such diverse activities as comparison shopping and political activism on legislation and other issues of vital interest to the disabled consumer.

Considering the fact that most clients are residents in transitional IL centers for only a few weeks or months, it is a tribute to the professionalism of the staffs of these centers that so many services can be provided. It should be remembered that all of these skills are being taught in addition to the daily provision of room and board and all the related services that these entail.

Goodwill Industries has developed a program resembling those of transitional IL centers to meet the needs of people who are less severely disabled than the usual transitional residence client, but are still in need of help because of their low incomes and semi-independent status (Laurie, 1977). This is an example of the kind of innovation and diversification in IL models by the private sector that is needed if the many disabled citizens still unreached by the rehabilitation movement are to be served.

## LONG-TERM INDEPENDENT LIVING CENTERS

There is no clear-cut division between those programs we have classified as transitional and those labeled long-term. For example, the Courage Center near Minneapolis has both a transitional residence component for clients still in training and a long-term residential component for clients who have entered employment at the center (Laurie, 1977). The primary distinctions between transitional and long-term residential centers involve the expected length of client participation and the goal of the services provided. Whereas short-term transitional programs concentrate on basic skills for social reentry, long-term residential programs usually have more severely disabled clients and seek to provide more complete training in a broader range of service areas. Long-term residential programs are also more likely to offer vocational training programs or evaluations. Other differences in the two types of centers will become clearer as specific examples are considered.

### SERVICES PROVIDED

The spectrum of services offered by long-term IL centers is even broader than that of the transitional centers. It ranges from infirmary care to halfway houses, with some centers, such as the Woodrow Wilson Rehabilitation Center in Virginia, offering services touching both ends of that continuum (Laurie, 1977). Since many of the services provided by long-term programs are similar to those already discussed under transitional programs, emphasis will be given here to the distinguishing features of long-term IL centers.

**Personal Skills**  Training in functional skills is provided to all clients, usually under the supervision of an occupational therapist and after a thorough individual evaluation has been performed. Medical rehabilitation is often provided in long-term centers by their own staff physicians and nurses, while psychological counseling for personal or adjustment problems is available from staff professionals as well as peer counselors. Some centers, such as the Lakeshore Rehabilitation facility in Birmingham, have hospital wings and can accept acute medical cases, whereas other centers require a relatively stable physical condition prior to entry (Laurie, 1977). Long-term residential centers teach medical and hygienic self-care as a way of reducing client medical costs and promoting good health. To assist the disabled person in maintaining a healthy lifestyle, information and instruction are provided concerning laundry and cleaning, nutrition, food buying, and the planning and preparation of meals. Just prior to the client's release, most long-term residential centers will send an occupational or physical therapist to the future home to evaluate its suitability for the client and to recommend changes.

**Social Skills**   Instruction in independent transportation is available in long-term residential centers, with some facilities even having driving simulators for increased safety while one is learning to use the adaptive equipment (Laurie, 1977). On-site and community recreation activities are extensive, frequently being planned and coordinated by a staff recreation director. Clients are taught to be their own advocates and to deal effectively with community agencies in preparing for their move into society. Each resident is trained in locating and obtaining appropriate housing, including instruction in the financing of a private home or the lease or rental of an apartment, and the planning of necessary accessibility adaptations. If necessary, the center staff will assist the disabled client with selecting an acceptable roommate, so that maximum cooperation and compatibility of needs is considered.

**Business-Related Skills**   During the extended time that each client spends in a long-term IL center, more in-depth instruction in business and management skills is given than in a transitional center program. For example, instead of the center merely providing a register of personal care attendants, the disabled person is taught to locate and train his or her own attendant. Since the attendant is individually trained by the disabled employer, the special needs and preferences of that employer can be easily accommodated. Being a competent trainer of attendants, the disabled person no longer requires highly specialized attendants

(Laurie, 1977). In fact, one's health and safety are more secure in the event of an emergency, because anyone who is available can be used to provide temporary assistance. Other matters, such as financial planning and daily activity scheduling, are also taught in more detail. However, the most significant factor affecting the future lifestyle of most clients is the presence of a variety of vocational training and employment options. In some centers, the training is similar to on-the-job or sheltered workshop programs, while in others it follows more traditional vocational instruction methods. With regard to employment, some centers have mostly assembly-line–type employment, while others employ clients in the center's kitchen, laundry, giftshop, or other facilities. Most programs incorporate some combination of these models, providing even more diversity. Long-term IL centers with a substantial number of elderly clients sometimes establish a "foster grandparents" babysitting service for the community, which provides the elderly residents with both financial rewards and social contacts (Caldwell and Hegner, 1975).

## GROUP HOMES

Group homes define independence as group living in a community setting (Cole, 1979). Although they were originally designed for mentally retarded and developmentally disabled people, group homes have proven useful for some physically handicapped people as well. One of the early government studies (completed in 1966) found that orthopedically handicapped adults placed in foster homes in the community had a much greater chance of becoming employed. This fact, and the reduced costs of community-based care, gave impetus to the group home movement for physically disabled people. Now some facilities, such as Handicap Village in Iowa, include both physically and mentally handicapped people with good results. The scope of group homes today is very broad, ranging from the one-month residential training and respite care of Marlborough House in Saint Louis to the many permanent residential facilities throughout the United States (Laurie, 1977). The size of group homes varies from single buildings that once were individual residences to clusters of cottages or buildings sharing central service and recreational facilities. In order to simplify the discussion of typical group home services, single unit homes and the larger programs will be considered separately.

## SINGLE-UNIT GROUP HOMES

There are two basic types of small group homes—those run by a landlord or manager and those operated by the residents themselves. In the traditional group home model, adapted from the system used with mentally retarded adults, the owner converts a large home into a boarding-house arrangement, but with modifications to ensure accessibility to the disabled tenants. Services usually provided include meals, recreational equipment and activities, limited transportation, general counseling, and houseparent-type assistance and supervision. There are rules about acceptable conduct, and each resident has particular duties such as cleaning his or her own room and washing his or her own laundry, in addition to assisting with the regular cleaning and maintenance of the common areas of the house. The owner helps clients with arranging and meeting required medical or therapy appointments, as needed. Such a program provides most of the security and other advantages of institutional care, but allows relative freedom in interactions with the community. The support of other residents and the owner often makes independent living in a small group home an attractive alternative for disabled people who would be at risk if living alone. While more active disabled people might consider the limited supervision and close tenant relationships of a small group home an intrusion on their privacy, these are small inconveniences, and sometimes even positive benefits, to a person who would otherwise be institutionalized.

The other type of small group home is one owned or rented by the disabled tenants themselves and operated on a cooperative or communal basis. Before moving into the home, several disabled people who are interested in sharing a house have gotten together, frequently with the assistance of a local IL center, and discussed their individual needs and desires. The center staff serves as a resource system in helping locate and evaluate the potential residents and residences. Through consultation either with the center's legal adviser or other legal services, the future owners or renters of the group home establish the legal rights and financial obligations of each person. Although somewhat less formal, this process is similar to establishing a business partnership.

Prior to occupancy, each disabled person makes a list of the services he or she requires and the times at which they must be performed. These services may include transportation to work or appointments, various types of therapy, help with bathing or bowels, dressing assistance, cooking, cleaning, or a multitude of similar activities. Either by themselves or with the advice of an IL center staff member, the group compiles all of these lists. Since the purpose of sharing a group home is to reduce costs and increase efficiency, mutual exchange of services among disabled residents is the first choice in obtaining assistance with individual needs. Any service needs that cannot be met by other residents are then consolidated in order to reduce the number of personal care attendants that must be hired and the number of trips made to accomplish necessary community contacts. A third alternative often used in obtaining personal care assistance is the provision of room and board to one or more nondisabled people in exchange for specified attendant services to the disabled residents. For full-time attendants, the room and board is supplemented with a salary.

An example of a group home that is owned by the disabled residents is Project Independence, which was purchased by a group of disabled young adults in Saint Paul, Minnesota, in 1972 (Laurie, 1977). The building was a four-unit apartment building that was converted to one large apartment downstairs and two small units upstairs. With gifts and the proceeds from fundraising benefits helping to start the project, most of the renovation was done by volunteers. In 1975 the residents moved in, occupying the 10-room apartment and renting the smaller ones to help meet the mortgage payments. The building is in a nice neighborhood and is served by a United Cerebral Palsy van, which provides transportation to work. There is a daytime housekeeper who cooks and cleans. Two student attendants are paid a salary in addition to being given free room and board in the house.

## CLUSTER-STYLE GROUP HOMES

When one hears the term "cluster housing" it should be remembered that the clustered units may be cottages, individual apartments, or apartment buildings. The key elements identified with the cluster housing concept of independent living, as compared to most small group homes, are: a larger number of residents, the provision of attendant, rehabilitation, and recreational services, and the offering of vocational training and employment opportunities to disabled residents. In contrast to the temporary nature of even long-term residential IL centers offering similar services, the large group homes are often places of permanent residence for disabled people. This does not mean, however, that mere custodial care is provided, since most homes offer a range of medical, therapy, or rehabilitation services to residents. Consideration of a few typical programs will illustrate the atmosphere and operation of cluster-style group homes.

**Cottage Programs** This category includes programs that are composed of a group of small cottages in a subdivision or resort colony arrangement. Each cottage is usually rented to one or two disabled people. Residents work in the yard and the garden, do housecleaning and maintenance, and help with other chores. Recreation is provided primarily on-site, but trips are made into town for shopping, church attendance, hair care, and so on. Food is purchased jointly for all residents and they participate in the buying, preparation, and serving of it. The cottage programs most resemble small group homes, except that some vocational training (mainly on-the-job training) and work opportunities are provided. Physical, occupational, speech, or other types of therapy are available at extra cost, as is transportation in some cases.

Two examples of successful cottage programs are Freedom Gardens for the Handicapped, Inc., in Lake Mohegan, New York, and Handicap Village in Clear Lake, Iowa (Laurie, 1977). Freedom Gardens has been in operation for twenty years and has ten apartment cottages located on five acres of land. It is more or less a housing project for disabled people but has attendants available for a fee and provides a communal recreation room. Handicap Village, on the other hand, has about 140 staff members and 150 residents, usually with 16 residents per cottage. They have a mixture of mentally and physically handicapped people, with the mentally retarded residents providing strength and attendant services and the physically disabled people acting as supervisors for activities on occasion. The residents do all they can for themselves, as the staff believes it is better to learn from failure than to be overprotected and never learn to be independent. Facilities are available for activities such as ceramics, crafts, music, gymnastics, and swimming.

**Apartment Cluster Programs** Because of their larger number of residents, comprehensive services, and permanence of residents, most apartment cluster programs have a friendly, supportive atmosphere resembling that of a small town. This environment is a positive influence on the individual's potential for independence in that it provides each disabled resident with a ready-made group of peers who know and care about one another (Milofsky, 1980). Some apartment cluster group homes are primarily concerned with the physical comfort and social and recreational needs of residents, placing less emphasis on training or employment. For example, the McLean Home in Connecticut has three levels of residential care, ranging from fully independent living to constant medical supervision. The home contains occupational, physical, and speech therapy rooms as well as clinical facilities. The McLean Home is designed around a central activity center, and interaction with the community is encouraged by a policy of inviting the town's residents to use the center for activities and cultural events. The program also has a day care center and recreational activities, although its primary emphasis is on rehabilitation of the residents (Laurie, 1977). Apartment clusters of another type concentrate on vocational evaluation, rehabilitation, employment training, and work programs for disabled adults. Some of their clients eventually move into the community to live and work, while the group home employs others in providing services after their training is completed.

Apartment cluster programs of a third type operate their own businesses to help support the cost of the residential facility while giving clients an opportunity for employment (Laurie, 1977). The Occupational Home and Apartments in Walworth, Wisconsin, operate a feeder cattle business that serves just such a purpose. Since its early days, when it was a camping program, the facility has expanded to include a gift shop, an indoor pool, a therapy wing, a workshop, and a picnic patio, as well as continuing the camping program. Job training and work opportunities are provided in other areas besides farming, including office work and phone answering and various duties in the gift shop. Transportation is provided for a fee, and interaction with the community is encouraged—especially church attendance, since the Occupational Home program is sponsored by a nondenominational religious organization. Most apartment cluster group homes provide recreational facilities and equipment, social facilities and activities, attendant and nursing care as needed, meals, and laundry facilities. Most resident needs can be met without having to leave the grounds of the facility. In a few cluster programs, such as the Creative Handicaps, Inc., apartment units in Houston, the project was established by disabled people themselves primarily to provide reasonable housing, shared attendants, and transportation (Laurie, 1977).

**Life Care Facilities**  The life care center is usually an apartment cluster facility also, but is specially designed for elderly disabled people (Caldwell and Hegner, 1975). Usually these buildings are equipped with intercoms, smoke and fire alarms, and security guard protection to enhance the safety and peace of mind of the residents. Ramps, automatic doors, and other accessibility features are standard. Social services offered include communal recreation areas and equipment, entertainment, group tours, lectures, and arts and crafts classes, to mention a few. Customary medical services are health and information referrals, infirmary care, temporary nursing care, and occupational or physical therapy. Training is given in ADL skills and the use of prostheses, with regular progress checks. Financial planning, and occasionally even vocational training, are available.

Traditional life care programs charge a monthly fee for all services, including maid service, meals, linens, and shopping trips to nearby stores at regular intervals. Some newer programs, however, are being established on a condominium-style plan where the elderly person buys a unit while still able to function independently and can live there knowing that a separate building housing medical and therapy services is available when the need arises. Tennessee has just given approval for a privately financed condominium-style development called Kirby Pines Estates, to be located in Memphis. This retirement complex for 600 people will have 416 apartments, with a 60-bed skilled nursing care center in an adjacent building ("Retirement Center," 1982). Life care facilities are frequently built by churches or civic organizations such as the Jaycees and, when the rental plan is used, a few units are often reserved for rental by people of lower income groups. The condominium units are also priced at various levels to accommodate different incomes, needs, and tastes. Residents are encouraged to remain as active as possible. Facilities are usually convenient to public transportation and community activities, with some programs even having their own vans or buses.

## SUMMARY

Each of the types of residential IL programs discussed in this chapter is better suited to some disabled people's needs than others'. Transitional programs are most beneficial to those who are not too recently disabled or who are able to return to their jobs but need personal care instruction. Long-term programs, on the other hand, allow adequate time for a lengthy recovery period and complete vocational retraining, if necessary. Both of these types of facilities are concerned with promoting maximum rehabilitation and returning the disabled client to independent residence in the community. Group homes, however, generally serve people who have reached almost maximum recovery and cannot, or do not wish to, live alone in the community. Valuable assistance with the establishment and orderly operation of group homes, especially small resident-owned ones, is regularly provided by local IL centers, thus benefitting both the disabled person and the community. The typical group home allows the resident less privacy than a private residence or apartment, but it provides many important benefits. In addition to the group home's facilities, there is the communal atmosphere and emotional support of staff and peers and the security of prompt medical support when an emergency arises. Before choosing any of these residential programs, a thorough evaluation by the disabled person of his or her abilities, goals, and physical and emotional needs is mandatory. The growing concern of elderly people for physical security and medical care as their health and mobility decline is creating a demand for life care and retirement centers with the appropriate services to care for them. This type of development is proving attractive enough to interest private investors and contractors, which bodes well for its future expansion.

# PART FOUR

*Assessing the Outcome*

# 13

## Determinants of Success and Failure

The ILR services paradigm described in this text is still an emerging concept. It does not yet have a proven track record, and the professionals who are struggling to prove its values and worthiness face the frustrations and the challenges of being pioneers in a new field. They do not have an established body of knowledge or panel of experts to whom they can turn for help when they encounter questions for which they have no answers and problems for which they can find no solutions. They are at the cutting edge of a rehabilitation movement entering new fields of endeavor. They are the experts in this field, and they are creating the body of knowledge they need.

As these professionals proceed to provide IL services to increasing numbers of elderly and disabled people, they will inevitably encounter failure with some, perhaps many, of their clients. These early failures are especially frustrating because there is so little research-based knowledge available to help prevent them, but they can also serve a useful purpose by calling attention to two important questions: (1) What accounts for the success or failure of ILR clients? (2) How can the chances for success be increased? The current ILR programs are, no doubt, already facing these questions.

These questions of success or failure are certainly not novel, as any experienced human service worker could testify. Even in service areas of long duration, no sure ways have been discovered to predict which clients will be successful and which will fail. In some cases certain categories of clients have been identified as having either high or low success rates, but even these categories provide little help in individual cases. If a prospective client in hypothetical category X is in counselor Jane's office, and counselor Jane knows that approximately 20 percent of the clients in category X succeed while 80 percent of them fail, then counselor Jane has the difficult question still before her. Is this particular client destined to be one of the 20 percent or one of the 80 percent? She probably does not have a clue to the answer of that question. Furthermore, counselor Jane has probably had many long coffee breaks during which she wondered why one client failed even after having received the highest quality rehabilitation services and why another succeeded in the face of overwhelming difficulties. These questions of success and failure have been the subject of much research in the more traditional rehabilitation disciplines. No doubt the same will be true in ILR.

The purposes of this chapter are to

1. review the more important factors that may influence success or failure in IL,

2. explore the importance of individual motivation to success,

3. describe an expectancy theory model as one that is especially useful in understanding motivational issues,

4. suggest steps that IL services staff members can take that can increase motivation and thus the chances for success.


## SUCCESS OR FAILURE: WHAT DOES IT MEAN?

In order to discuss the factors that influence success or failure it seems necessary to clarify what would be considered success and what failure. Traditionally, discussions of success or failure in rehabilitation literature have focused upon clients achieving success in reaching rehabilitation program goals (Kir-Stimon, 1978; Roessler, 1980). This means that the rehabilitation program espouses certain goals as being desirable and valuable, and the program's staff attempts to help clients achieve those goals. For example, Kir-Stimon (1978), in discussing research studies that explore the success or failure of rehabilitation clients, noted that success was "measured by end-employment or some life-productive task" (p. 189). One must assume that if a client did not achieve employment or life-productivity as defined by the rehabilitation program then that client would not be judged successful, even if he considered himself successful in achieving the goals most important to him. In other words, rehabilitation success has been measured in terms of the degree to which clients achieve rehabilitation program goals, not necessarily client goals.

The measurement of success as just described is understandable and justifiable in light of the nature of rehabilitation programs. For example, the vocational rehabilitation program of each state is funded for the express purpose of improving the employability of disabled people. What better measurement of program success could there be than a determination of how effectively that program helps disabled people to return to work? If a disabled person wants to avail himself or herself of the services of the vocational rehabilitation agency, then he or she must understand that those services are designed and funded for that specific goal of employability; and if his or her personal goals do not include employment, then, unfortunately, he or she is simply outside the target population served by that agency.

Given their clearly delineated goals in the past, the measures of success for rehabilitation agencies, while not perfect, have at least been clearly understood. In the newly established ILR programs, success may be much more difficult to define and measure. As noted in earlier chapters, IL is an ambiguous concept, which, at best, can be understood as a continuum that ranges from the abstraction of complete dependence to the abstraction of complete independence. If an individual was at point $X$ on that continuum and has moved forward to point $Y$, is that individual successful or unsuccessful? That depends upon whether he or she has the physical, mental, and emotional capacity to move beyond point $Y$, whether he or she has the external support services and other resources to move beyond point $Y$, and whether he or she wants to move beyond point $Y$.

In addition to the fact that IL must be measured in terms of degrees along a continuous scale, ILR programs are responsible for addressing client needs in the broadest possible range of life areas. This complicates matters considerably. Earlier rehabilitation programs, such as medical rehabilitation or vocational rehabilitation, were able to focus their efforts on achieving specific goals. While it was necessary to address issues from all areas of life, still the program staff could address those issues in terms of their effect upon a primary program goal such as physical functioning or employment. ILR programs, on the other hand, have no one focal area of most importance. If the client's needs are primarily physical, then that becomes the focal point of the IL program. If the client's needs are financial, are in the housing area, are emotional, or whatever, then that area of need becomes the focal point of the IL program. This is an unprecedented challenge in the rehabilitation field, and it is as much a challenge in measuring success as in meeting such a broad array of needs.

Roessler (1981) proposes a method by which ILR programs may evaluate success. He suggests that results be measured in the areas of physical functioning, economic independence, psychosocial development, educational functioning, and vocational functioning. The degree of functioning in each area can then be measured and compared with some standard to determine success. This procedure of breaking down the IL program into more manageable and measurable areas of functioning is necessary if one is to have any chance at all of measuring success in a reasonably effective manner.

While proposals such as Roessler's should work quite effectively in providing a methodology for measuring success, they perhaps gloss over the basic issue raised at the beginning of this discussion. What does success really mean in IL? If one says that success in IL is equal to the sum of the successes in the various areas such as physical functioning, vocational functioning, or psychosocial development, then the basic question is simply redirected to those areas. What then determines success in physical functioning and the other areas pertinent to IL? Roessler's proposal suggests that success in those areas be measured by specific instruments. For example, physical functioning could be measured by an instrument like the IL behavior checklist (Walls et al., 1979). The effect of measuring success in this way is that ultimately success in physical functioning (or other areas being measured) is determined by the client's ability to do those things that the instrument measures. This leaves the IL program staff in a position where the definition of success is caught in an endless loop. That is, an instrument becomes both the tool used to measure success and the definition of success.

It may be impossible to avoid completely this problem of the instrument having an influence on the definition of success. At least one important step, however, can be taken to lessen that influence. In developing the IL plan with each individual client, the goals specified in the plan should be carefully delineated to represent accurately what the client wants to achieve. Once the goals are well defined, an appropriate instrument to measure progress toward those goals can be sought. As Roessler (1981) suggests, carefully specified goals may offer clear, objective means of measurement in themselves.

Achievement of the goals specified in the individualized written IL program is perhaps the best definition of success in IL. If success is defined in this way, then the IL process becomes a client-centered process in which what the client perceives as desirable and as possible becomes the goal and the central focus of the plan of action. This sets the ILR program apart from all other rehabilitation programs, in which the success of clients must be determined by their achievement of the program's goal.

## SUCCESS OR FAILURE: WHAT MAKES IT HAPPEN?

Given that success in IL is an individualized concept that is determined by the degree to which an individual client achieves his or her IL goals, what factors are responsible for that success? Since ILR programs are so recent in origin, there is not yet enough research evidence to answer that question definitively. Nevertheless, research done in earlier rehabilitation programs should reveal some factors related to success that are also applicable in IL. Some of the factors identified as important to rehabilitation success are self-concept, self-esteem, age, extent and nature of disability, previous work history, education, and motivation (DeLoach and Greer, 1979; Kaplan and Questad, 1980). Some of these factors—work history, for example—are probably less important in ILR than they are in vocational rehabilitation, but others—such as motivation, for example—may be just as important, or even more so.

Of the factors listed as important to success, some are outside the client's control (for example, extent of disability) while others are within the client's control (for example, self-concept, self-esteem, and motivation). If one can influence the client's chance for success by somehow influencing those factors, then it is helpful to know which factors can be influenced by the client himself and which require the intervention of some other person. In this same vein, it is interesting to note that there is no factor in the list that would not have an influence upon the final factor, motivation. Furthermore, motivation may well be the most important of all factors. DeLoach and Greer (1979) review research studies in which rehabilitation counselors indicate that they perceive client motivation as the most critical variable in rehabilitation success. If counselors so consistently believe motivation to be critically important to rehabilitation success, then it likely is an important factor, if only because of the tendency for prophecies to be self-fulfilling. Since motivation is an important factor, and one that may be influenced by a number of other client variables, it will be included as a key element in this discussion of factors influencing success in IL.

## CLIENT MOTIVATION

Motivation is often used to convey a variety of meanings. It may be used to imply that an individual is in readiness for a task (as in "he is motivated to play well"), to describe something done to another person (as in "that counselor motivates his clients"), or to "refer to a quality possessed by an individual" (as in "she is a person with motivation") (Wilkins and Alexander, 1981, p. 138). In common usage the term motivation is used with so many different meanings and to account for so many different phenomena that it almost becomes meaningless. In this discussion, however, motivation will be used to discuss why ILR clients may choose to act or not act, and why they choose particular goal-directed actions from among the many goal-directed actions available to them (Kelly, 1958).

Several motivation theorists (McClelland, 1961; Maslow, 1954; Murray, 1962) postulate that people's actions are in response to experienced needs. The actions chosen by the individual are those actions that he or she perceives as having the potential to reduce an experienced need. This explanation of motivation may be applicable in ILR, since clients typically are involved in this process because they have needs that require outside assistance. However, the concept of need is so commonly understood to mean a deficit, or something lacking, that this explanation of motivation, while it may be technically correct, seems insufficient to account for some actions that are intended to add even more to the individual's life rather than to compensate for something missing.

Expectancy theory is an explanation of motivation that is clear and simple to understand, and it is not subject to the shortcomings of the need theories. This theory has been developed primarily in the fields of industrial psychology, organizational theory, and management as a means of exploring work motivation. It states that, first, "people have preferences among the various outcomes available to them. Second, people have expectancies about the likelihood that effort on their part will lead to the desired behavior or performance. Third, people have expectancies about the likelihood that certain outcomes will follow their behavior. Finally, in any situation, the actions a person chooses to take are determined by the expectancies and the preferences that the person has at that time" (Wilkins and Alexander, 1981, p. 138, based on Lawler, 1973). For example, an ILR client may consider living in his own apartment a very desirable outcome. He may expect that if he puts forth effort he will acquire the personal care, homemaking, and cooking skills necessary to maintain his own apartment. He may also expect that, as a result of acquiring the skills necessary to maintain an apartment and acquiring the income necessary to pay the rent, he will rent and live in his own apartment. Given his expectation that he can acquire certain skills and income, his expectation that acquiring those skills and income will result in his being able to rent an apartment, and his preference for his own apartment as an outcome, then his actions will likely be directed toward getting that apartment.

This expectation that effort will lead to the desired behavior or performance is called performance expectancy (sometimes referred to as $E_1$). The expectation that certain outcomes will follow the desired performance or behavior is called outcome expectancy (sometimes referred to as $E_2$). And the preference for a specific outcome among many available outcomes is called valence. Motivation to act depends upon all three of these components being present. Had the client in this example not valued the idea of having his own apartment, then that outcome would not have enticed him to action. But even if he valued that outcome highly, if he had not expected that effort on his part would enable him to achieve the outcome, then he would not have been motivated to act. Finally, if he had perceived some other way as the easiest route to the desired outcome instead of the actions mentioned, he could have followed that course of action. For example, he might have perceived getting his own apartment as being dependent upon his getting enough financial disability benefits to hire a full-time attendant. If so, his objective would have been to try to get that level of disability benefits rather than to take actions that would lead to an increased level of ADL skills and income.

A description of the steps involved in motivation is only a part of the story. Given that motivation is an important element in successful IL, it becomes important to consider what factors influence motivation and success, and what actions can be taken by IL professionals to increase the client's motivation and, consequently, the client's chances for success.

## FACTORS THAT INFLUENCE
## MOTIVATION AND SUCCESS

**Family**    Probably the most important of all the external factors contributing to the ultimate success of the disabled individual is the family. The family can place real barriers before the disabled individual and can undermine his belief in his ability to succeed. On the other hand, the family can remove barriers and can inspire the disabled person to lofty achievements.

The family can influence the disabled or elderly person's motivation at the point of both performance and outcome expectancy. Lawler (1973) says that performance expectancy is influenced by past experience, the actual situation, self-esteem, and feedback from others. The family may influence the individual's performance expectancy in any of these ways but especially in providing feedback. The family may be a primary reference group for a disabled or elderly person, and the feedback the individual gets from his family will be very important to him in shaping his performance expectancy. Much has been said about the overprotective parents, for example, whose relationship with their disabled child communicates to him that if he attempts too much he will surely fail (Dunham, 1978). By the time he is grown up, this type of fearful attitude, though understandable, can have the disabled person convinced that no amount of effort on his part could possibly lead to successful performance. Such overprotective attitudes are not limited to parents of disabled children. Elderly parents sometimes feel stifled when around their grown children, who believe that since their parents are old they must be getting too weak and too senile to take care of their business, their homes, and themselves without help.

The effect of family overprotectiveness is to communicate to the disabled person that he is incompetent to perform in a multitude of ways. This attitude, if it is internalized by the disabled person, serves to lower his self-concept and his performance expectancy. If, later, he has an opportunity to become involved in an ILR program, the person will be unmotivated—not because independence as an outcome or goal is unattractive but because the person does not believe that he can perform at the level required to make independent living possible.

A second way that the family can influence motivation is by altering the individual's perception of the linkage between performance and outcome. As stated earlier, a person will be motivated to a specific action for a highly desirable outcome only if he or she perceives that outcome as being contingent on that action. Often family members are guilty of promising a treat to a disabled family member as a reward for performing a certain task, but then later giving the reward even though the task was not performed. For example, parents might promise a disabled child an ice cream cone after dinner if he manages to eat his dinner without assistance, but then give the child the ice cream cone even though he did not eat his meal without assistance. They might do so because the child is crying and they feel sorry for him, because he is angry and says they are unfair, or because they think he tried, even though unsuccessfully, to eat without assistance. Assuming that it is within the ability of the child to eat without assistance and assuming that this is a consistent pattern of behavior, then the child is learning that the outcomes he desires are not necessarily contingent upon competent performance. Instead those desired outcomes may just as easily be obtained by crying or pouting, by expressing anger at perceived unfairness, or even by "gallantly trying" though without success.

This type of experience is detrimental to the motivation of the disabled person. When confronted with the usual rewards available in life, the person whose outcome expectancy has been altered in this way may look for a way to receive the rewards without meeting the challenges. Clearly, this is often impossible when one is finally forced to leave the protective world of the family, and thus the person's misdirected motivation will likely lead only to frustration and failure. Bates (1977) describes an effective training program to teach parents or other family members how to avoid such problems. Behavioral principles are used with parents in order to teach them how they can use behavioral principles themselves with their disabled child.

Of course not all influence from families is negative. There are certainly many families who are supportive of their disabled members without being overprotective, and who can allow their disabled members their personal independence without completely abandoning them. The support that families are uniquely capable of giving can have a beneficial influence on the disabled person's self-concept, performance expectancy, and eventual success. Because families can make such an important contribution to rehabilitation, many writers have suggested that the family be actively involved in the rehabilitation process. Bray (1980) suggests that families be included in the rehabilitation process as service recipients just as the disabled person is. Services rendered to families would include counseling, communication training, training and assistance in problem solving techniques, family contracting, and assertiveness training. Such attempts to involve the family in the rehabilitation process can improve the contributions that this most important resource makes to the disabled person.

**Past Experiences** A second factor that influences the individual's motivation and success is the cumulative effect of past experience. Conventional wisdom says that the best predictor of future success is past performance. In the case of ILR, past experiences may mean the success with which the individual has coped with his disability, or it may mean the degree to which the individual lived successfully before becoming disabled.

Two examples from familiar cases illustrate the effect of past experience quite clearly. Two of the example cases introduced in Chapter 2 and referred to many times in this text are Eleanor M. and Marie S. The cumulative effect of past experiences upon Eleanor is highly positive. Eleanor has had an independent spirit all her life. She has attempted a wide range of activities in her life and has experienced some measure of success in all of them. She has not avoided failure in all cases, but on those occasions where she did fail she was able to learn and profit from the experience. Thus, she was able to transform failures into learning opportunities, and as a result she rarely felt the deep emotional reactions of self-doubt and depression that often accompany the experience of failure.

Marie, on the other hand, has a long history of avoiding any attempts to stretch her potential. She has seldom attempted any meaningful activity at which she has been able to experience the joy of succeeding. Her past failures have influenced the way she perceives herself so that she will see herself as a failure in almost any situation. If she were to attempt a new task and complete 75 percent of it successfully, she would likely believe she had failed because she did not complete all of it. She would feel, emotionally, like a failure even though there is just as much, or even more, reason to feel successful. Often people such as Marie need to be taught how to see the success in their lives. Otherwise the experience of failure will continue to dominate them unreasonably.

The motivational effect of past experience in the case of Marie and others like her is to lower the person's performance expectancy to the point where she is not motivated by any outcomes, no matter how highly valued they might be. The ILR staff can take at least two steps to intervene in such a situation. They can guide the client in reevaluating past experience in order to find the successes as well as the failures, and they can begin developing new success experiences.

In reevaluating past experiences, the counseling staff should find the rational-emotive therapy of Ellis (1973) quite useful. This counseling approach demands that the person look at external events in an objective fashion and realize that his emotional reactions are caused not by the events themselves, but by his beliefs about those events. This provides a perfect framework for exposing what may often be irrational perceptions of failure in past experiences. Thus the client may not be able to change his past, but he can certainly change the way he perceives his past and the way he feels about it.

The other suggestion for intervention is that the staff of the IL program help the client to begin experiencing success in as many ways as possible. It is important to remember that the client may not perceive success readily, and therefore experiences may need to be devised in which quick and obvious success is almost certain. The staff can also point out success in process to the client. This entails reassuring the client who is involved in a process leading to an eventual goal that while he has not yet achieved the ultimate goal, he has successfully completed some of the steps necessary to achieve that goal.

Role playing is one excellent way of building these initial success experiences. The role-playing situation can be arranged in the security of the counselor's office or some other appropriate place. The topic can be one that the client will eventually have to deal with in the real world. Finally, the situation itself can be rehearsed as many times as necessary to ensure success. In settings of this kind, the client can experience success in process and success in final performance and can rehearse for success in the world. If structured properly, role playing can even be an effective training tool for nondisabled IL staff members, family members, or others involved in the IL process (B. A. Wright, 1978).

**Negative Incentives**   One of the most frustrating factors influencing success or failure is the list of negative incentives with which disabled and elderly people and their families must contend. Negative incentives are the result of flukes in public program policies that make it more advantageous for a disabled or elderly person to remain dependent than to become independent. People who are disabled may receive direct financial compensation from a number of different sources, including Social Security Disability Insurance (SSDI), Supplemental Security Income (SSI), Workers' Compensation, private long-term disability insurance, and veterans' benefits (Eaton, 1979; Schlenoff, 1979; Walls et al., 1977). In addition, a number of other valuable benefits are available, such as assistance with education, job training, housing, food stamps, and medical care. The sum total of all financial assistance being received by a disabled person is often much more than that person could earn at a job if he were working.

The financial disincentive to become economically independent by working is one of the most commonly cited negative incentives, but there are other important examples. Pieper and Cappucilli (1980) discuss the policies of many state agencies, which allow them to financially subsidize the care of a disabled or elderly person in a total care institution but will not allow them to subsidize that person at home, even at less cost to the state. The case of Susan J., discussed in Chapter 2, illustrates well the dilemma facing many disabled people and their families. Because her family's income is considered adequate by the state, even though it is in the lower-middle income range, Susan is not eligible for many of the medical and financial benefits offered by the state. The state would, however, place Susan in an institution and pay the entire cost of her being there. The irony is that the state could help the family provide for Susan at home for as little as one-tenth the cost of placing her in an institution. Thus, some disabled people, who would otherwise like to achieve greater independence in the community, choose the more dependent situation because it is all they can afford.

Safilios-Rothschild (1970) adds to the financial disincentives already mentioned the psychological disincentives of the secondary benefits of disability and dependency. Discussion of concepts such as secondary benefits and the sick role may well be describing the effect that the many incentives to dependency have on the motivation of the individual to become independent. The disabled or elderly person may believe that effort on his part will lead to the level of performance necessary for IL, but he finds that if he does perform at that level, the outcomes are not what he expected. Instead of gaining a life of more freedom and dignity, he loses vital medical and economic benefits. As a result he learns that if he is to maintain those benefits that are important to his survival he must choose dependence rather than independence. In effect, he is motivated to be dependent.

With the other factors that influence success or failure, intervention steps have been suggested that can lessen the negative effects and can take advantage of the positive effects of those factors. Unfortunately, the intervention steps needed to deal effectively with negative incentives are beyond the power of the IL staff members or clients to take. These financial disadvantages are the result of the policies that guide the action of public agencies. The only really effective way to change this situation is to change the laws and the policies. People involved in ILR can attempt to bring about such changes by communicating their concerns and their suggestions to legislators, congressmen, and public agency administrators.

**Individual Characteristics** Success or failure is also influenced by such things as the severity of the person's physical, mental, and emotional restrictions, the initial level of his skills, his financial resources, and the quanity and quality of support services available to him. Some people are caught in dependency situations that are simply overwhelming while others are fortunate in having a wealth of assistance to help them become independent.

With more than ten million severely disabled people in the United States, even if only a small percentage were caught in severely restricting circumstances, there would still be a large number of people needing help. There is evidence that there are many people in such circumstances, especially in rural areas where services are not available and where transportation is a problem. Cook et al. (1981, p. 56) estimate that "approximately 5,000,000 handicapped individuals live in towns of 2,500 or less." The lack of accessible services, community resources, and opportunities can make independence difficult for these people, many of whom are severely disabled. Add to this the number of disabled and elderly people in urban areas who have similar problems, and the number of people caught in severely restricting circumstances becomes extremely significant.

Severely restricting circumstances obviously have an effect on motivation and success. If a person is severely disabled, is denied access to ILR services because of distance or some other reason, and has few personal resources on which he can rely, the motivational result will be the destruction of any belief on the part of the individual that he or she can become independent. Again it matters little how attractive an outcome such as independence might be. For an outcome to be motivational, the individual must perceive it as attainable.

For people caught in circumstances such as these, ILR programs can mean the difference between success and failure. The services available through the state/federal ILR programs are especially well suited to filling these gaps in service availability. In designing their individualized plans to meet specific client needs, it is important that the staff and the client carefully assess both the situational variables and the client's personal abilities. If this assessment reveals that the client actually has the ability already to overcome at least some of the problems facing him, this will be a motivational boost for him and will give a good start to the IL plan. Of course such a careful assessment also has the additional advantage of providing the accurate information needed to develop an effective plan of action.

IL programs also need to offer improved and expanded services in order to be of greater benefit to those caught in disadvantageous circumstances. There is evidence that rehabilitation professionals themselves believe that they already have the capacity to meet client needs more effectively than they are doing. Walton et al. (1980) found a significant gap between the degree to which certain techniques and concepts are perceived by rehabilitation professionals as important in IL and the degree to which they are actually used in the field. Such discrepancies must be eliminated for ILR programs to be as effective as possible in helping promote the motivation and the success of severely disabled people.

ILR programs also need to expand if they are to be able to meet the needs of those who are not being served at present. In many places IL services are still not available because existing programs serve only a limited geographical area. Most existing IL programs are funded through Part B, Centers for Independent Living, of Title VII of the 1978 Rehabilitation Amendments. Part B was the only portion of the IL provisions initially funded. It is designed to offer services through centers for IL, which necessarily limits the geographical area that can be served. The full funding and implementation of Part A, Comprehensive Services, could alleviate this situation by offering comprehensive IL services to virtually every area of the country.

**Other External Factors** The most obvious factors influencing motivation and success are the family, past experiences, negative incentives, and situational variables. There are, however, a number of other factors external to the individual that also can influence motivation and success. In fact, one could argue that all interactions between an individual and his environment influence his motivation to some extent. Some interactions, however, are more important than others. For the disabled or elderly person who is attempting to become independent, environmental barriers, both physical and emotional, may have a significant effect on motivation.

In Chapter 8 the importance of community accessibility to IL was discussed. A community with inaccessible public buildings and public transportation can severely hamper an individual with mobility impairments, and those accessibility problems can reduce his motivation just as much as they reduce his mobility. A community that does not make itself accessible to disabled people literally shuts the door in their faces. It communicates to the disabled or elderly citizen that he is not wanted or needed as a part of the community. This, in turn, affects the disabled or elderly citizen's perception of his chances to be independent. For some the effect may be minimal, but for others it will convince them that their efforts toward independence are futile. They feel they will never be a part of the community anyway.

Other interactions with the environment involve not physical barriers but emotional ones. In many subtle ways, as well as many not so subtle, the disabled and elderly have been treated as less than equal in this society. An example is the way disabled and elderly people are spoken to and spoken about. The language of this society includes many terms and phrases used in reference to disabled and elderly people that convey negative attitudes about them, and the way disabled and elderly people have been portrayed in the mass media has conveyed a similar message. Even though in recent years there has been much improvement in this area, there are still disabled and elderly people in society who have lived with negative attitudes and prejudice for years. Some of those people have less motivation to try to succeed in their communities because of their emotional reactions to the attitudes of others.

An important part of the environment for disabled and elderly people is the part occupied by physicians and other rehabilitation professionals. The attitudes of professionals toward disabled and elderly people have long been a problem (DeLoach and Greer, 1981), and especially so for the motivation of the individual. Many professionals have responded to their disabled clients with an attitude that seems to focus on the disability rather than on the many residual abilities and skills the person still has. Professionals often are not aware of the true potential of their clients, and they make decisions and suggestions about treatment and other action programs that leave the client functioning well below his real capacity. As one can easily imagine, unrealistic expectations and attitudes from professionals carry over into reduced client effort toward goals that he has been led to believe are not attainable.

The most effective way to combat community barriers, negative attitudes and prejudice, and unrealistically restrictive professional attitudes is through education and advocacy. ILR programs can do much to correct mistaken beliefs by implementing community education programs. These programs can be especially effective when they highlight the active involvement and accomplishments of severely disabled and elderly people in the community. The IL staff can also serve as advocates for any person having difficulty in overcoming negative attitudes or prejudice in a particular business, agency, or individual. Community education and advocacy are perhaps as important as any service provided by IL programs.

**Internal Factors**  All the factors previously mentioned that influence motivation and success are external to the individual. Each of those factors, however, affects the disabled person's self-concept, his motivation toward IL, and ultimately his chances for successful IL. As mentioned above their influence is as much a result of their psychological effect on the individual as of the external restrictions they place upon him. Individually and collectively they have a serious effect on the person's belief that he is capable of competent performance and that competent performance will result in the desired outcome of IL. As the individual is affected in this way, he gradually develops the expectation that he cannot perform and that even if he does perform, he still will not attain the goals he desires. In essence, the individual has become motivated to fail. He expects to fail, and he does fail.

In discussing each of the factors that influence the person's motivation, intervention steps were suggested that can lessen the harmful effects of those factors. The purpose of those interventions is to break the cycle in which the individual lowers his expectations because of the influence of external factors, fails in his intended performance, and then attributes his failure to the external factor rather than to his own lowered expectations. Research evidence indicates that a person who believes that he can influence his environment is more likely to be an effective performer than one who believes that his environment dominates him (Currie-Gross and Heimbach, 1980). Furthermore, the individual's perception of the locus of control can be influenced by effective counseling and training. The client can learn to exert control over those external factors affecting his life.

## SUMMARY

This chapter has discussed the concept of success and the factors that influence success in ILR. Since success is determined by the client's achievement of planned goals, the definition of success in IL differs from that of earlier rehabilitation programs. In an IL program, the goals specified are for each client and represent what the client wants to accomplish in his life. In a vocational rehabilitation program, on the other hand, the program goal—for example, employment—is the same for all clients. Since client goals and program goals in ILR are virtually the same, success is truly a client-centered concept in this program.

In this chapter client motivation has been presented as a critically important determinant of success or failure. An expectancy theory model of motivation has been presented as a useful tool in understanding and thus in influencing and facilitating, client motivation. This model of motivation suggests that people are motivated to action when they value a particular objective and expect that effort on their part will lead to desired performance, which, in turn, will lead to the valued outcome.

Several factors that can influence motivation and success have been discussed. The effect that these factors can have on the client's motivation has been clarified, and intervention steps have been suggested that can help to make this effect beneficial rather than harmful.

Perhaps the greatest contribution that IL services will make to their clients is that they will help them to have a chance to succeed or to fail. Some people probably will fail, but failure is not disgrace. Failure may even offer an individual an opportunity to learn and mature that would not be available in any other way (Mottershead, 1977). In every endeavor, some people will succeed immediately, and still more will fail along the way toward eventual success. The severely disabled and elderly people who are involved in ILR programs are not different from the rest of the population. Some have made it. Some have not. And some are still on the way.

# References

Anderson, M. 1977. Power to the crips. *Human Behavior* 6:48–49.

Are polios getting older faster? 1981. *Accent on Living* 26(3):30–37.

Aronson, R. 1976. The role of an occupational therapist in a geriatric day hospital setting. *American Journal of Occupational Therapy* 30:290–292.

Barrier free design. 1975. United Nations expert group meeting on barrier free design. *Rehabilitation International*, June 1975. Monograph.

Bates, P. 1977. The search for reinforcers to train and maintain effective parent behaviors. *Rehabilitation Literature* 38:291–295.

Baum, C. 1980. Independent living: A critical role for occupational therapy. *American Journal of Occupational Therapy* 34:773–774.

Benedict, R. C., and Ganikos M. L. 1981. Coming to terms with ageism in rehabilitation. *Journal of Rehabilitation* 47(4):10–18.

Berkson, G., and Romer, D. 1981. A letter to a service provider. In: H. Haywood and Z. Newbrough (eds.), *Living Environments for Developmentally Retarded Persons*. Baltimore: University Park Press.

Berman, E. 1978. *The Solid Gold Stethoscope*. New York: Ballantine.

Bitter, J. A. 1979. *Introduction to Rehabilitation*. St. Louis: C. V. Mosby.

Blake, R. 1981. Disabled older Americans: A demographic analysis. *Journal of Rehabilitation* 47(4):19–27.

Bolton, B. 1981. Assessing employability of handicapped persons: The vocational rehabilitation perspective. *Journal of Applied Rehabilitation Counseling* 12:40–44.

*Boston Center for Independent Living* (BCIL). Undated. (Informational brochure.)

Bowe, F. 1978. *Handicapping America: Barriers to Disabled People.* New York: Harper & Row.

Bowe, F. 1980. *Rehabilitating America: Toward Independence for Disabled and Elderly People.* New York: Harper & Row.

Bozarth, J. O. 1981. The rehabilitation process and older people. *Journal of Rehabilitation* 47(4):28–32.

Bray, G. P. 1980. Team strategies for family involvement in rehabilitation. *Journal of Rehabilitation* 46(1):20–23.

Brearly, C. P. 1977. *Residential Work with the Elderly.* London: Routledge and Kegan Paul.

Brickner, P. W., Janeski, J. F., and Duque, T. 1976. Hospital home health care program aids isolated, homebound elderly. *Hospitals* 50 (1 November 1976):118–120, 122.

Brotman, H. B. 1976. Every tenth American: The "problem" of aging. In: M. Lawton, R. Newcomer, and T. Byerts (eds.), *Community Planning for an Aging Society: Designing Services and Facilities.* Stroudsburgh, Pa.: Dowden, Hutchinson, & Ross.

Bruck, L. 1978. *Access.* New York: Random House.

Caldwell, E., and Hegner B. R. 1975. *Geriatrics.* Albany, N.Y.: Delmar Publishers.

Cappaert, A. 1979. Confusing definitions of independence. *Rehabilitation Gazette* 22:25–26.

Carp, F. M. 1976. Urban livestyle and life-cycle factors. In: M. Lawton, R. Newcomer, and T. Byerts (eds.), *Community Planning for an Aging Society: Designing Services and Facilities.* Stroudsburg, Pa.: Dowden, Hutchinson, & Ross.

Cary, J. R. 1978. *How to Create Interiors for the Disabled.* New York: Pantheon Books.

Cobb, A. B. (ed.). 1973. *Medical and Psychological Aspects of Disability.* Springfield, Ill.: Charles C Thomas.

Cole, J. 1979. What's new about independent living? *Archives of Physical Medicine and Rehabilitation* 60:458–462.

Cook, D., Ferrito, D., and Cooper, P. 1981. A challenge for the 1980's: Rehabilitating the rural disabled. *Journal of Rehabilitation* 47(2):56–59.

Currie-Gross, V., and Heimbach, J. 1980. The relationship between independent living skills attainment and client control orientation. *Journal of Rehabilitation* 46(2):20–22.

*Daily Herald,* Wausau, Wisc., 30 July 1981.

Dart, J., Dart, Y., and Nosek, P. A philosophical foundation for the independent living movement. *Rehabilitation Gazette* 23:16–18.

DeJong, G. 1979. The movement for independent living: Origins, ideology, and implications for disability research. Paper presented at the American Congress of Rehabilitation Medicine, 17 November, New Orleans, La.

DeJong, G., and Wenkler, T. 1979. Attendant care as a prototype independent living service. *Archives of Physical Medicine and Rehabilitation* 60:477–482.

DeLoach, C., and Greer, B. G. 1979. Client factors affecting the practice of rehabilitation counseling. *Journal of Applied Rehabilitation Counseling* 10(2):53–59.

DeLoach, C., and Greer, B. G. 1981. *Adjustment to Severe Physical Disability: A Metamorphosis.* New York: McGraw-Hill.

Deyoe, F. S., Jr. 1972. Spinal cord injury: Long-term follow-up of veterans. *Archives of Physical Medicine and Rehabilitation* 53:523–529.

Dowd, E. and Emner, W. 1978. Lifeboat counseling: The issue of survival decisions. *Journal of Rehabilitation* 44(3):34–36.

Dunham, C. S. 1978. The role of the family. In: R. M. Goldenson, J. R. Dunham and C. S. Dunham (eds.), *Disability and Rehabilitation Handbook.* New York: McGraw-Hill.

Dunn, D. J. 1981. Vocational rehabilitation of the older worker. *Journal of Rehabilitation* 47(4):76–81.

Eaton, M. W. 1979. Obstacles to the vocational rehabilitation of individuals receiving workers' compensation. *Journal of Rehabilitation* 45(2):59–63.

Edgerton, R., and Bercovici, S. 1976. The cloak of competence: Years later. *American Journal of Mental Deficiency* 80:485–497.

Ellis, A. 1973. Rational-emotive therapy. In: R. Corsini (ed.), *Current Psychotherapies.* Itasca, Ill.: F. E. Peacock Publishers Inc.

Equal access not so easy for buses, subways. *U.S. News and World Report*, 20 July 1981, p. 45.

Ferleger, D., and Boyd, P. A. 1980. Antiinstitutionalization: The promise of the Pennhurst Case. In: R. J. Flynn and K. E. Nitsch (eds.), *Normalization, Social Integration, and Community Services.* Baltimore: University Park Press.

Fiedler, L. 1978. *Freaks: Myths and Images of the Secret Self.* New York: Simon and Schuster.

Flemming, A. S. 1972. A national policy to maximize independent living for older people. In: C. Osterbind (ed.), *Independent Living for Older People.* Gainesville, Fla.: University of Florida Press.

Flint, W., and DeLoach C. 1975. A parent involvement program model for handicapped children and their parents. *Exceptional Children* 41:556–558.

Flynn, R. J., and Nitsch, K. E. 1980. Normalization: Accomplishments to date and future priorities. In: R. J. Flynn and K. E. Nitsch (eds.), *Normalization, Social Integration, and Community Services.* Baltimore: University Park Press.

Frieden, L. 1977. Community and residential based housing. In: *White House Conference on Handicapped Individuals, Volume One: Awareness Papers.* Washington, D.C.: U.S. Government Printing Office.

Frieden, L. 1980. Independent living models. *Rehabilitation Literature* 41:169–173.

Geist, C. S. 1980. Development of an independent living rehabilitation program curriculum. *Journal of Rehabilitation* 46(2):53–55.

Gilbert, A. E. 1973. *You Can Do It from a Wheelchair.* New Rochelle, N.Y.: Arlington House Publishers.

Gives, V. M. 1978. Financial aid and special services. In: R. M. Goldenson, J. R. Dunham, and C. S. Dunham (eds.), *Disability and Rehabilitation Handbook.* New York: McGraw-Hill.

Golant, S. 1979. *Location and Environment of Elderly Population.* Washington, D.C.: V.H. Winston & Sons.

Gold, M.W. 1975. Vocational training. In: J. Wortis (ed.), *Mental Retardation and Developmental Disabilities: An Annual Review,* Vol. 7. New York: Brunner Mazel.

Goldenson, R. M., Dunham, J. R., and Dunham, C. S. (eds.). 1978. *Disability and Rehabilitation Handbook.* New York: McGraw-Hill.

Goodkin, H. F. 1977. Transportation accessibility. In: *White House Conference on Handicapped Individuals, Volume One: Awareness Papers.* Washington, D.C.: U.S. Government Printing Office.

Gorski, R. 1981. Is the Barriers Board heading for a last hurrah? *Disabled USA* 4:7–9.

Greenstein, D., Gueli, C., and Leonard, E. 1976. No one at home. *Rehabilitation Literature* 31:2–9.

Hale, G. 1979. *The Sourcebook for the Disabled.* New York: Paddington Press.

Hamilton, K. 1950. *Counseling the Handicapped in the Rehabilitation Process.* New York: Ronald Press.

Harwell, J. 1980. A primer on using HUD programs. *Challenge* 11(11):10–11.

Hasselkus, B., and Kiernat, J. 1973. Independent living for the elderly. *American Journal of Occupational Therapy* 27:181–188.

Heal, L. W., Sigelman, C. K., and Switzky, H. N. 1980. Research on community residential alternatives for the mentally retarded. In: R. J. Flynn and K. E. Nitsch (eds.), *Normalization, Social Integration, and Community Services.* Baltimore: University Park Press.

Hirschberg, G. G., Lewis, L., and Vaughn, P. 1976. *Rehabilitation: A Manual for the Care of the Disabled and Elderly.* Philadelphia: J.B. Lippincott.

Hitz, R. 1980. Living alone. *Rehabilitation Gazette* 23:19–20.

Howse, J. L. 1980. Piecing together existing financial resources. In: P. Roos, B. M. McCann, and M. R. Addison (eds.), *Shaping the Future: Community-based Residential Services and Facilities for Mentally Retarded People.* Baltimore: University Park Press.

Huttman, E. D. 1977. *Housing and Social Services for the Elderly.* New York: Praeger Publishers.

Hylbert, K., Sr., and Hylbert, K., Jr. 1979. *Medical Information for Human Service Workers.* 2nd Ed. State College, Pa.: Counselor Education Press.

Hylbert, K., Sr., and Hylbert, K., Jr. 1981. *Medical Information for Human Service Workers.* 3rd Ed. State College, Pa.: Counselor Education Press.

Independent Living Research Utilization Project (ILRUP). 1979. *A Technical Assistance Manual on Independent Living: Sourcebook.* Houston: Institute for Rehabilitation and Research.

International Labour Office. 1973. *Basic Principles of Vocational Rehabilitation of the Disabled.* 2nd Ed. Geneva: International Labour Office.

*J. C. Penney Company Catalog.* Fall and Winter, 1981.

Jameson, F. 1981. The great wheelchair controversy. *Reader's Digest,* August, pp. 11–16.

Kaplan, M. 1981. Vocational follow-up: Physically restored unemployed SCI. *SCI News Briefs,* pp. 1, 3.

Kaplan, S., and Questad, K. 1980. Client characteristics in rehabilitation studies: A literature review. *Journal of Applied Rehabilitation Counseling* 11:165–168.

Katz, D., and Kahn, R. L. 1978. *The Social Psychology of Organizations.* 2nd Ed. New York: John Wiley & Sons.

Kelly, G. 1958. Man's construction of his alternatives. In: G. Lindzey (ed.), *Assessment of Human Motives.* New York: Holt, Rinehart, and Winston.

Kerr, N. 1972. Staff expectations for disabled persons: Helpful or harmful. *Rehabilitation Counseling Bulletin* 14:85–94.

Kiernat, J. 1976. Geriatric day hospitals. *American Journal of Occupational Therapy* 30:285–288.

Kir-Stimon, W. 1978. Psychodynamics in rehabilitation of the physically disabled. *Rehabilitation Psychology* 25:187–194.

Kleinfield, S. 1979. *The Hidden Majority.* Boston: Little, Brown.

Knight, A. 1980. Attitudinal, social, and legal barriers to integration. In: P. Roos, B. McCorn, and M. Addison (eds.), *Shaping the Future: Community-Based Residential Services and Facilities for Mentally Retarded People.* Baltimore: University Park Press.

Kolstoe, O. P., and Frey, R. M. 1965. *A High School Work Study Program for Mentally Subnormal Students.* Carbondale, Ill.: Southern Illinois University Press.

Kutner, B. 1971. Rehabilitation: Whose goals? Whose priorities? *Archives of Physical Medicine and Rehabilitation* 52:282–287.

Lampos, C. 1981. Achievement. *National Voice of the Disabled,* December, p. 9.

Lancaster, J. 1976. Testimony before the Senate Subcommittee on the Handicapped of the Committee on Labor and Public Welfare. *Paraplegia News* 29:32–34.

Laurie, G. 1975. A compendium of employment experiences of 101 quadriplegics. *Rehabilitation Gazette* 18:2–26.

Laurie, G. 1977. *Housing and Home Services for the Disabled.* New York: Harper & Row.

Laurie, G. 1980. Respiratory rehabilitation and post-polio aging problems. *Rehabilitation Gazette* 23:3–11.

Laurie, G. 1981. (Editorial.) *Rehabilitation Gazette* 28:2–3.

Laurie, G., and Laurie, J. 1976. A compendium of employment experiences of 21 more quadriplegics. *Rehabilitation Gazette* 24:15–20.

Lawler, E. E. 1973. *Motivation in Work Organizations.* Monterey: Brooks/Cole.

Leeds, M. Housing directions for the elderly. 1973. In: R. Davis (ed.), *Housing for the Elderly.* Los Angeles: University of Southern California.

Lenihan, J. 1977. Disabled Americans: A history. *Performance.* Washington, D.C.: President's Committee on Employment of the Handicapped.

Lifchez, R., and Winslow, B. 1979. *Design for Independent Living.* New York: Whitney Library of Design.

McClelland, D.C. 1961. *The Achieving Society.* Princeton, N.J.: Van Nostrand.

McDaniel, J. W. 1976. *Physical Disability and Human Behavior.* 2nd Ed. New York: Pergamon Press.

Mace, R. L. 1977. Architectural accessibility. In: *White House Conference on Handicapped Individuals, Volume One: Awareness Papers.* Washington, D.C.: U.S. Government Printing Office.

McGowan, J. F., and Porter, T. L. 1967. *An Introduction to the Vocational Rehabilitation Process.* Washington, D.C.: U.S. Department of Health, Education, and Welfare, Vocational Rehabilitation Administration.

McKinley, J. B. 1975. Who is really ignorant—physician or patient? *Journal of Health and Social Behavior* 16:3–11.

Maguire, G. 1979. Volunteer program to assist the elderly to remain in home settings. *American Journal of Occupational Therapy* 33:98–101.

Mallik, K., and Mueller, J. 1975. Vocational aids and enhanced productivity of the severely disabled. In: *Devices and Systems for the Disabled.* Krusen Center for Research and Engineering at Moss Rehabilitation Hospital.

Margolin, R. J. 1971. Motivational problems and resolutions in the rehabilitation of paraplegics. *American Archives of Rehabilitation Therapy* 20:95–103.

Maslow, A. H. 1954. *Motivation and Personality.* New York: Harper.

Matlack, D. 1975. The case for geriatric day hospitals. *Gerontologist* 15(4):109–113.

May, E., Waggoner, N. R., and Hotte, E. B. 1974. *Independent Living for the Handicapped and Elderly.* Boston: Houghton Mifflin.

Milofsky, C. 1980. Serving the needs of disabled citizens. *Social Work* 25(2):149–152.

Moakley, T., and Weisman, J. 1981. Cost: Is the price of accessible mass transit too high? *Paraplegia News* 35:46–49.

Mitchell, P. 1976. *Act of Love: The Killing of George Zygnarik.* New York: Alfred A. Knopf.

Mottershead, C. V., Jr. 1977. A chance to fail. (Editorial.) *Rehabilitation Literature* 38, inside front cover.

Murray, H. 1962. *Explorations in Personality.* New York: Science Editions.

National Center for Health Statistics. 1977. *Vital and Health Statistics.* Series 13, Number 32. December.

Newcomer, R. J. 1976. Meeting the housing needs of older people. In: M. Lawton, R. Newcomer, and T. Byerts (eds.), *Community Planning for an Aging Society: Designing Services and Facilities.* Stroudsburg, Pa.: Dowden, Hutchinson, & Ross.

Nirje, B. 1969. The normalization principle and its human management implications. In: R. Kugel and W. Wolfensberger (eds.), *Changing Patterns in Residential Services for the Mentally Retarded.* Washington, D.C.: President's Committee on Mental Retardation.

Nirje, B. 1980. The normalization principle. In: R. Flynn and K. Nitsch (eds.), *Normalization, Social Integration, and Community Services.* Baltimore: University Park Press.

Novick, L. 1973. Day care meets geriatric needs. *Hospitals* 47:47–50.

Obermann, C. E. 1965. *A History of Vocational Rehabilitation in America.* Minneapolis: T. S. Denison & Co.

Office of Information and Resources for the Handicapped, U.S. Department of Education. 1980. *Programs for the Handicapped.* January/ February. Washington, D.C.

Office of Information and Resources for the Handicapped, U.S. Department of Education. 1981. *Programs for the Handicapped.* May/June. Washington, D.C.

Palmore, E. B. 1972. Measuring the quality of life among the elderly. In: C. Osterbind (ed.), *Independent Living for Older People.* Gainesville, Fla.: University of Florida Press.

Parameter, T. R. 1980. *Vocational Training for Independent Living.* International Exchange of Information in Rehabilitation. New York: World Rehabilitation Fund.

Parsons, T. 1958. Definitions of health and illness in the light of American values and social structure. In: E.G. Jace (ed.), *Patients, Physicians, and Illness.* Glencoe, Ill.: Free Press.

Payne, J. S., Mercer, C. D., and Epstein, M. H. (eds.). 1974. *Education and Rehabilitation Techniques.* New York: Behavioral Publications.

Pieper, B., and Cappucilli, J. 1980. Beyond the family and the institution: The sanctity of liberty. In: T. Apolloni, J. Cappucilli, and T. P. Cooke (eds.), *Achievements in Residential Services for Persons with Disabilities: Toward Excellence.* Baltimore: University Park Press.

Pratt, L., Seligman, A., and Reader, G. 1958. Physicians' views on the level of medical information among patients. In: E. G. Jace (ed.), *Patients, Physicians, and Illness.* Glencoe, Ill.: Free Press.

Provencal, G. 1980. The Macomb-Oakland regional center. In: T. Apolloni, J. Cappuccilli and T. P. Cooke (eds.), *Achievements in Residential Services, for Persons with Disabilities: Toward Excellence.* Baltimore: University Park Press.

Rabin, D. L. 1981. Physician care in nursing homes. *Annals of Internal Medicine* 94:126–127.

Ramsey, P. 1978. *Ethics at the Edge of Life.* New Haven, Conn.: Yale University Press.

Retirement center passes last hurdle. 1982. *Commercial Appeal,* 27 May 1982, pp. A1, A3.

Rice, B. D., and Roessler, R. T. 1980. *Introduction to Independent Living Rehabilitation Services.* Arkansas Rehabilitation Research and Training Center.

Richardson, S. A. 1972. People with cerebral palsy speak for themselves. *Developmental Medicine and Child Neurology* 14:524–535.

Roessler, R. T. 1980. Factors affecting client achievement of rehabilitation goals. *Journal of Applied Rehabilitation Counseling* 11:169–172.

Roessler, R. T. 1981. Program evaluation in independent living rehabilitation. *Journal of Applied Rehabilitation Counseling* 12:200–204.

Roessler, R. T., and Bolton, B. 1978. *Psychosocial Adjustment to Disability.* Baltimore: University Park Press.

Roosevelt Warm Springs Institute for Rehabilitation. 1982. *Annual Report.* Warm Springs, Ga.

Rose, E. A. 1978. *Housing for the Aged.* Westmead, England: Saxon House.

Ross, E. C. 1980. The evolution of HUD programs serving persons with disabilities: An outsider's perspective. *Challenge* 11(11):6–8.

Rubin, S., and Roessler, R. 1978. *Foundations of the Vocational Rehabilitation Process.* Baltimore: University Park Press.

Rusk, H. 1977. *Rehabilitation Medicine.* 4th Ed. St. Louis: C. V. Mosby.

Safilios-Rothschild, C. 1970. *The Sociology and Social Psychology of Disability and Rehabilitation.* New York: Random House.

Schlenoff, D. 1979. Obstacles to the rehabilitation of disability benefits recipients. *Journal of Rehabilitation* 45(2):56–58.

*Sears, Roebuck, and Company Home Health Care Catalog,* 1981.

Seventh Institute on Rehabilitation Issues. 1980. *Implementation of Independent Living Programs.*

Shaw, D. 1981. Showdown on Capitol Hill: Home health care legislation in the 80's. *Rx Home Care* 3:19–25.

Smith, C. 1977. Independent living experiences. *Housing and Home Services for the Disabled.* New York: Harper & Row.

Smith, N. K., and Meyer A. B. 1981. Personal care attendants: Key to living independently. *Rehabilitation Literature* 42:258–265.

Stanton, E. 1970. *Clients Come Last.* Beverly Hills, Cal.: Sage Publications.

Stein, J. 1978. *Making Medical Choices: Who Is Responsible?* Boston: Houghton Mifflin.

Stoddard, S., and Brown, B. 1980. Evaluating California's independent living centers. *American Rehabilitation,* November–December, pp. 18–23.

Swinyard, C. A., Menolascino, F. J., Taylor, E. J., Staros, A., Rubin, G., and LeClair, R. 1977. Rehabilitation and treatment. In: *White*

*House Conference on Handicapped Individuals, Volume One: Awareness Papers.* Washington, D.C.: U.S. Government Printing Office.

The accessible home. 1981. *Better Homes and Gardens Remodeling Ideas,* Fall, pp. 65–79.

Thorenson, R., Smits, S., Butler, A., and Wright, G. 1968. Counselor problems associated with client characteristics. *Wisconsin Studies in Vocational Rehabilitation,* Monograph no. 3. Madison, Wisc.: Regional Rehabilitation Research Institute.

Tidyman, E. 1974. *Dummy.* Boston: Little, Brown.

Trigiano, L. L., and Mitchell, J. 1970. Physical rehabilitation of quadriplegic patients. *Archives of Physical Medicine and Rehabilitation* 51:592–594, 613.

U.S. Congress. 1973. *Public Law 93–112, The Rehabilitation Act of 1973.*

U.S. Department of Transportation. 1976. *Urban Mass Transportation Act of 1964 and Related Laws.* Washington, D.C.

U.S. Department of Transportation, Transport System Center and Urban Mass Transportation Administration. 1973. *The Handicapped and Elderly Market for Urban Mass Transit, Executive Summary.* Washington, D.C., July.

Verville, R. E. 1979. Federal legislative history of independent living programs. *Archives of Physical Medicine and Rehabilitation* 60:447–451.

Vineberg, S., and Willems, E. 1971. Observation and analysis of patient behavior in the rehabilitation hospital. *Archives of Physical Medicine and Rehabilitation* 52:8–14.

Walls, R. T., Ma'sson, C., and Werner, T. J. 1977. Negative incentives to vocational rehabilitation. *Rehabilitation Literature* 38:143–150.

Walls, R. T., Zane, T., and Thvedt, J. 1979. *The Independent Living Behavior Checklist.* Morgantown, W. Va.: West Virginia Rehabilitation Research and Training Center.

Walton, K. M., Schwab, L. O., Cassatt-Dunn, M. A., and Wright, V. K. 1980. Independent living techniques and concepts: Perceptions by professionals in rehabilitation. *Journal of Rehabilitation* 46:57–63.

Weinberg, N., and Williams, J. 1978. How the physically disabled perceive their disabilities. *Journal of Rehabilitation* 44(3):31–33.

*Wheelchair II Conference Proceedings.* 1979. Washington, D.C.: U.S. Government Printing Office.

*White House Conference on Handicapped Individuals, Volume Three: Implementation Plan,* 1978.

Wilkins, R. D., and Alexander, E. R. III. 1981. Expectancy theory as an approach to the motivation of rehabilitation counselors. *Journal of Applied Rehabilitation Counseling* 12:138–142.

Williams, M. G. 1981. Independent living for older people. *Journal of Rehabilitation* 47(3):69–71.

Williams, R., and Benes, N. 1976. The day hospital. *American Journal of Occupational Therapy* 30:293.

Wolfensberger, W. 1972. *Normalization: The Principle of Normalization in Human Services.* Toronto: National Institute on Mental Retardation.

Wolfensberger, W. 1978. The ideal human service for a socially devalued group. *Rehabilitation Literature* 39:15–17.

Wolfensberger, W. 1980. A brief overview of the principle of normalization. In R. Flynn and K. Nitsch (eds.), *Normalization, Social Integration, and Community Services.* Baltimore: University Park Press.

*Word from Washington,* July 1981.

Wright, B. A. 1960. *Physical Disability—A Psychological Approach.* New York: Harper & Row.

Wright, B. A. 1978. The coping framework and attitude change: A guide to constructive role playing. *Rehabilitation Psychology* 25:177–183.

Wright, G. N. 1980. *Total Rehabilitation.* Boston: Little, Brown.

Young, J. S., and Northup, N. E. 1979. Statistical information pertaining to some of the most commonly asked questions about SCI—Part II. *SCI Digest* 1:11–27.

Young, J. S., and Northup, N. E. 1980. Re-hospitalization in years two and three following spinal cord injury. *SCI Digest* 2:21–34.

# Index

**267**